Medical Coding and Billing Fundamentals 2023

The Definitive Handbook to Launch a Prosperous Career in Medical Billing and Coding for a Promising Financial Future

Table of contents

Chapter 4: Medical Billing

Introduction

Someone must handle the insurance and patient billing, also known as medical coding, at every medical facility. Doctors or office managers may perform these chores in addition to their primary responsibilities, or they may be delegated to an employee or employees. Since clinical staff needs to focus on patient care, it is common practice to have trained professionals handle the crucial administrative work of coding and billing.

Coding and billing services for healthcare transform patient encounters into the vocabulary of claims and compensation.

Providers can't get paid for their services without going through the two distinct but interrelated steps of billing and coding.

Billing patients and submitting insurance claims requires the use of medical codes. On the other hand, medical coding refers to the process of extracting billable information from a patient's medical record and clinical documentation. The creation of claims is the hub of the healthcare revenue cycle, where medical billing and coding meet.

The procedure begins with the patient signing up and concludes when the provider is paid for all services rendered. The time it takes to complete the medical billing and coding cycle varies from a few days to several months, depending on the nature of the services provided, the effectiveness of the organization's claim denial management, and the frequency with which patients are required to pay their bills.

Having a well-trained medical billing and coding team can help healthcare companies run more efficiently, allowing doctors and other employees to receive full reimbursement for their high-quality treatment.

Chapter 1: What is medical billing and coding

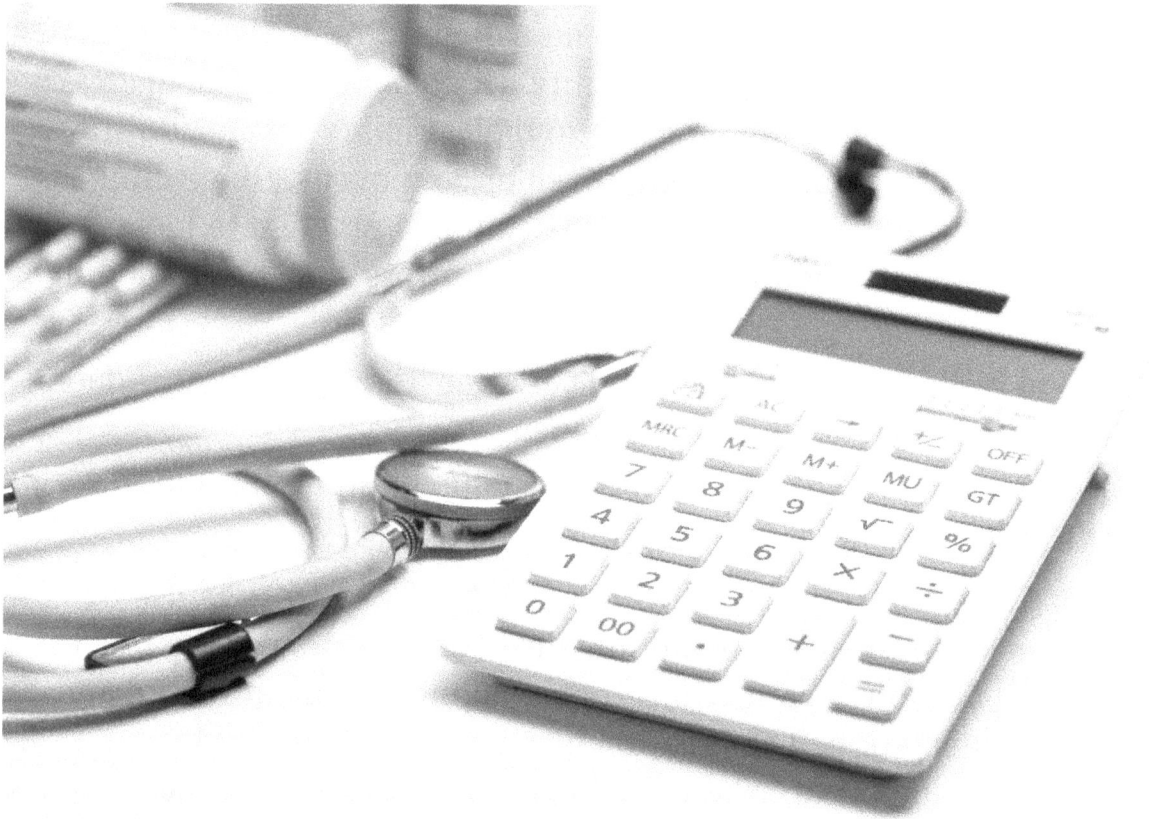

Medical billing and coding are used to submit and process insurance claims so that the healthcare practitioner will eventually get paid.

Without a medical biller and coder, paying for healthcare services would be a significant nuisance and create issues within an office. Therefore, this position is crucial to the healthcare business. Hospitals, doctors' offices, healthcare facilities, commercial insurance companies, and government-owned corporations are all potential employers for medical billers and coders. They are charged with managing the billing cycle and cash flow of their place of business.

Medical billers and coders organize patients' medical information into formats accepted by insurance companies to guarantee that healthcare providers get reimbursed. There is no distinction between medical coding and billing regarding average pay. The most significant elements affecting earnings are the employer, geography, and years of experience.

Medical coders use the three primary code sets, CPT, ICD, and HCPCS, to assign codes to each component of a patient's care. Because medical records are intricate, coding is a form of shorthand that condenses the principles to make the billing process more accessible. Billers in the medical industry use the codes to generate invoices for patients and insurance companies. Billers' work guarantees that healthcare providers get compensated. Depending on your employer and the company size, you might undertake both coding and billing tasks or specialize in one or the other. Coders and billers primarily use numbers in their work. Accuracy is essential since even a minor error can prevent the insurance company from making a payment.

Did they think about computer coding vs. medical coding? They differ from one another. Medical coders and billers use computers, but they are entering codes that have been developed and defined for the healthcare sector. Coding is utilized in the development of websites, applications, and software programs in a large number of businesses.

Chapter 2: differences between coding and billing

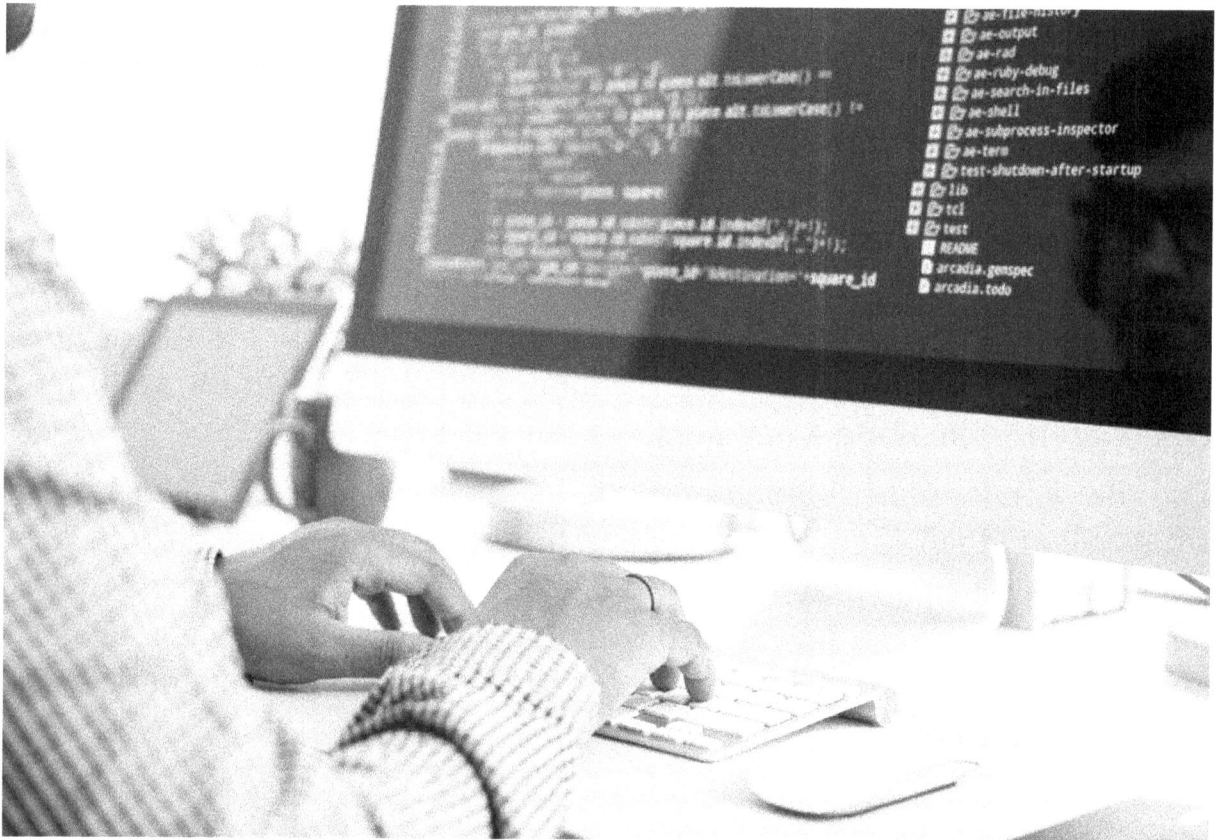

Medical coding and billing are two separate responsibilities, although most believe they are equivalent job duties. These two tasks could appear identical to the layperson, yet they have some significant distinctions. Professionals in these industries use similar abilities to produce comparable outcomes, but their strategies and techniques differ.

Both professions require translating medical documents into standardized codes to transmit vital medical information to the appropriate people; hence these two skill sets overlap. The function of a medical coder is to offer the most detailed account possible of a medical encounter. The billers are responsible for handling the financial aspects of the contact. Medical billers, on the other hand, are responsible for providing accurate and timely reimbursement based on the codes.

What Medical Billers Do

Medical billers oversee using patient data and coded claims to send invoices for provided treatments to various insurance carriers. In contrast to medical coding, which often does not include direct patient contact, this function frequently involves interpersonal engagement. Medical billers collaborate with patients, insurance providers, and other parties to guarantee that all payments are completed correctly and swiftly. Medical billers must be thoroughly aware of the range of medical language, the insurance policies of medical providers, and several insurance companies.

Once the codes are in the system, medical billers utilize medical billing software to create a claim.

They converse with patients, medical staff, and insurance companies in charge of making payments.

The billing specialist will likely be the one to contact the insurers for a guarantee of payment if authorization from an insurance carrier is necessary before executing a service. They will follow up on past-due bills by contacting patients, sending claims to collection companies, and contesting rejected claims.

Billers will also discuss with patients their deductibles, copayments, and any other obligations based on their insurance plan.

Medical Coding Process

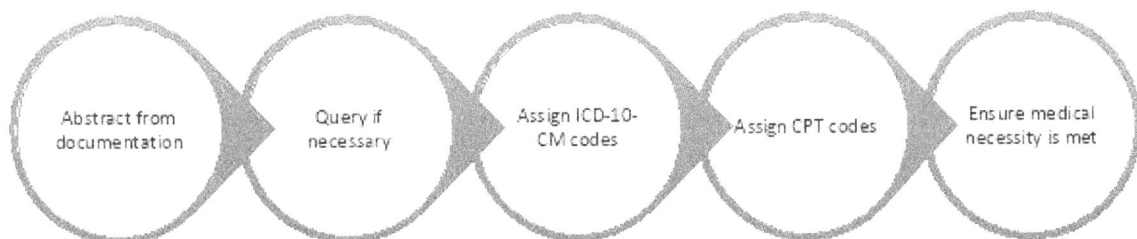

Abstract from documentation → Query if necessary → Assign ICD-10-CM codes → Assign CPT codes → Ensure medical necessity is met

What Medical Coders Do

Medical coders are in charge of transforming procedural information into quickly recognizable codes that insurance companies can understand and use to settle claims. To speed up the settlement of claims, various coding techniques are employed to establish the correct coding:

Current Procedural Terminology (CPT) - These codes are utilized for treatments in outpatient settings or doctors' offices.

In accordance with the Healthcare Common Procedure Coding System, these codes designate procedures that are covered by both Medicaid and Medicare (HCPCS).

ICD-9, or the International Classification of Diseases, is a set of designations used to describe various illnesses.

Coding professionals in the medical field are required to be experts in all coding methods. Together, medical billers and coders can support accurate claims that can be processed quickly.

In essence, medical coders describe what happened during a patient visit. They are responsible for examining the medical records the doctor has provided and converting the data into medical codes.

For instance, a doctor may check on a patient or may have prescribed an X-ray for a patient with an acute traumatic injury. Whatever the cause of the visit, each diagnosis, procedure, or service should be given a unique code to receive the correct compensation.

These codes are assigned based on the national categorization systems, and they can be input into computer software, handwritten notes, paper, and electronic files. They can also be assigned by hand.

A medical coder will use the ICD-10-CM, CPT, and HCPCS Level II categorization systems when documenting care provided in an outpatient setting. In inpatient settings, medical coders make use of both the ICD-10-CM and the ICD-10-PCS.

The medical necessity of a procedure, service, or supply provided to a patient is communicated to payers by reporting the appropriate codes based on the provider's paperwork. The coder must consult the physician or other staff members if there are any concerns regarding the documentation.

Chapter 3: Medical Coding

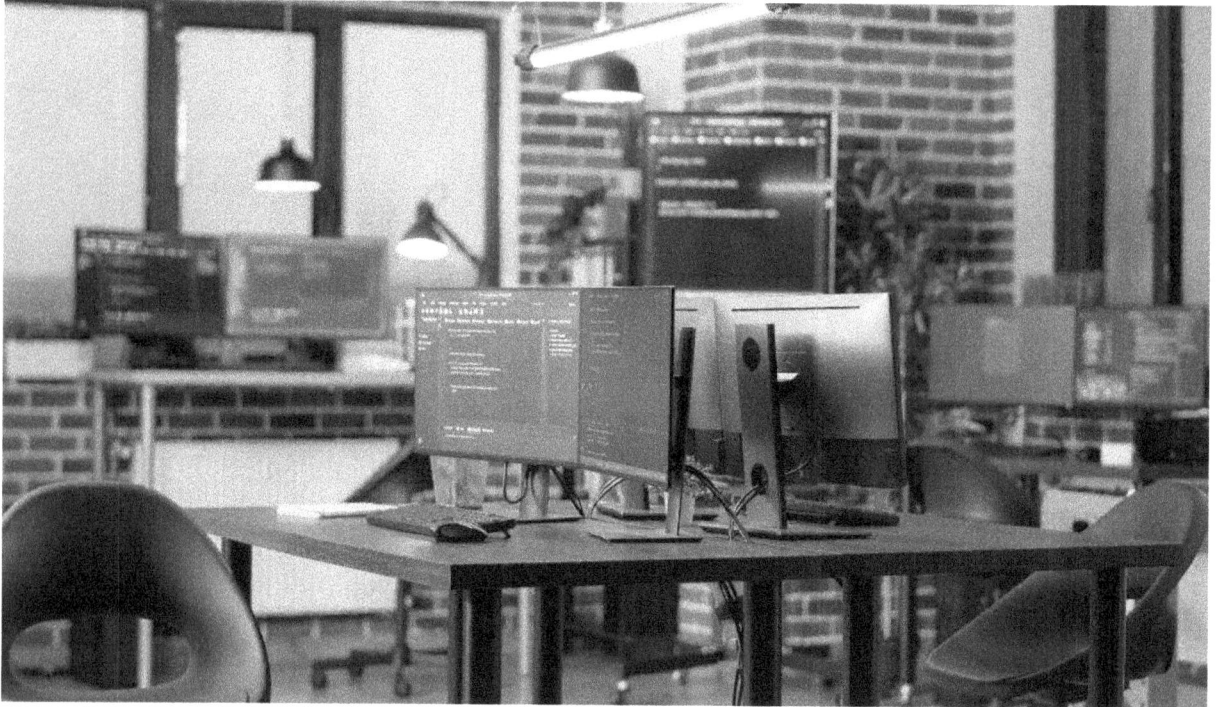

Medical Coder's task

Medical coding offers a standardized method for healthcare practitioners to maintain patient data and bill insurance companies. The payment process is now much more efficient than before this position was added. The payment method can become complicated because each provider and insurance company collaborates with dozens of other providers, governmental organizations, and insurance carriers. Errors can lead to complex solutions, denied claims, erroneous billing, and frustrated patients, all of which are detrimental to the patient in the long run. Medical coding was created to prevent just that. It now serves as a crucial component of healthcare, assisting with hospital reimbursement and patient insurance.

Medical Coder Responsibilities and Duties

- Enter the patient's insurance, referring physician, and demographic information in the medical management system.
- Take care of insurance authorizations and verifications.
- Talk to the office financial managers about referrals and insurance authorizations.
- According to business regulations, enter word codes into the medical management system.
- Follow check-and-balance procedures to ensure proper code capture.
- Make code additions or corrections in response to audit findings.
- Examine the latest Medicare bulletins and local coverage determinations.
- Maintain accurate records to support thorough coding and adhere to legal requirements.
- Maintained coding dictionaries, supervised version control, and adhered to it.
- Participate in local and international coding committees and provide tactical support for coding problems.
- Educate staff members on data coding.
- Work with data management and medical stakeholders to carry out coding rules and process procedures.
- To address unclassifiable codes, collaborate with the international coding committee.
- Create coding standards for knowledge about drug safety.
- Educate and train the user community in applying manual and automatic coding standards.
- Many individuals are under the impression that medical billing and coding are the same professions, however this is a common misconception. They are two distinct professions that different individuals often carry out in entirely different areas of a hospital, clinic, or doctor's office. Of course, one person could do practically everything in a tiny office.
- The graduates of the Andrews School's online medical coding training program are employed in various settings. Others work in clinics and doctor's offices, while some are used in hospitals. Those who work in

medical coding, nursing homes, and billing services for medical practices are employed by medical insurance companies. The duties shift depending on the kind of establishment as well as the level of certification held by the medical coder.

- To be qualified to apply for medical coding positions in any of those medical environments, coders must complete the Andrews School training program and get the highest level of professional coding credentials.
- Medical coders examine a patient's medical record to identify the patient's diagnoses and any operations that were carried out. They then classify those diagnoses and procedures following a national categorization scheme, giving each one a unique numeric or alphanumeric identifier.
- Put another way, a medical coder converts the written information in a patient's chart into codes. The coding specialist is a crucial healthcare team member and frequently provides information on documentation, rules, reimbursement, and data collecting for doctors, administrators, and other allied health practitioners.
- Coders may write code using computer software, fill in the blanks in handwritten notes, or employ a combination of paper and digital files on any given day. Every hospital, clinic, and doctor's office handles it differently.
- A professional coder must possess an in-depth understanding of anatomy and physiology, disease processes, pharmacology, the many classification systems, and more to effectively read a patient's chart and record the information therein.

Why Should You Think About Becoming a Medical Coder?

The employment of medical secretaries, including medical coders, is expected to increase by 22% between 2016 and 2026, which is substantially faster than the average for all professions, according to the U.S. Bureau of Labor Statistics (BLS). The positive job outlook may facilitate the availability of jobs for qualified coders.

The Bureau of Labor Statistics reported that the annual mean wage for medical secretaries was $34,610 as of May 2017, the most recent month for which data was available. On the other hand, gaining years of experience in the field in addition to a professional certification, such as the Certified Professional Coder (CPC®) accreditation offered by the AAPC, may result in higher wages. According to the findings of the 2017 AAPC Salary Survey, coders who had an average of 13 years of experience and the CPC certification earned a yearly salary of $54,106.

To begin a career in medical coding, you are required to have either a high school diploma, a General Equivalency Diploma (GED), or an equivalent. The next step is to obtain the necessary training, which usually entails enrolling in a school for medical coding. You can select a degree or diploma program and campus-based or online learning.

In a period of less than a year, it is possible to earn a certificate or diploma. On the other hand, completing the requirements for an associate's degree could take up to two years (both depending on the rate of the individual student). If you want to upgrade your qualifications or enroll in a bachelor's degree program in the future, an associate degree can be a good alternative for you. On the other hand, if you want to start looking for a career in medical coding right away, a diploma program might be a better option for you.

Some courses will prepare you to obtain a professional certification, like the CPC certificate. To become certified, you must pass an exam the certifying organization gives, meet specific eligibility requirements, and receive a passing score. For instance, in order to become a certified professional coder (CPC), you need to have either one year of work experience plus 80 contact hours from a coding preparatory school or two years of on-the-job training. Passing the exam grants new graduates the CPC Apprentice (CPC-A) designation, which can be upgraded to the full CPC with documentation of experience.

After graduating and obtaining your certification (if you so desire), you can begin looking for work as a medical coder in hospitals, doctors' offices, and other healthcare settings. Let's examine what your typical workday might entail.

Medical coder's methods for translating services and other services

Professional medical coders should be trained to understand and execute their job entirely. To use codes appropriately, they must have a thorough understanding of conventional medical codes and how they are used, as well as a mastery of how to read a patient's report. There are only a few of private training centers and schools that provide certification programs in medical billing and coding. In addition, you have the option of taking self-study courses either online or through the mail.

A trained specialist in coding carries out his professional responsibilities with a complete comprehension of the patient's medical file. Unique ideas and technical phrases are used to construct the medical language. When a doctor is writing a document for a patient meeting, the material that is relevant to the medical report needs to be accurate and precise. Together with doctors and other healthcare professionals, Coders can understand a patient's condition and course of treatment using specialist words.

Coding Audits

During the auditing process, a comparison is made between the documentation in the medical records and the codes that are present in the medical claims. This helps ensure that the codes are accurate. Either a medical institution preceding claim filing completes this task or a third party does. If submitted claims are not supported by thorough evidence, it may result in legal liability and charges of reimbursement fraud and abuse. Claims are presented with legal justification thanks to the professional and accurate coding work of a licensed and trained medical coder.

Federal government agencies and commercial health insurers routinely carry out claims audits. An expert in coding checked the medical report to ensure its accuracy, carefully examining the supporting documents.

Medical Abbreviations

Medical terminology frequently includes abbreviations. They facilitate speedier report documentation for doctors and other medical professionals. One abbreviation can have multiple associated terms, leading to misunderstandings or blunders. Therefore, it is crucial to use medical acronyms with caution. There is a lengthy list of these abbreviations, and getting the proper knowledge only comes from certified training.

Be familiar with the various medical terms

There are specific names for each of the anatomical structures that make up the human body. The technical names were created from words in Latin and Greek. By being aware of the definitions of various roots and affixes, multiple terms can be deciphered. There is a possibility that medical reports and records will contain terminology with Latin and Greek roots. They will be able to issue the proper code for the medical operation if they thoroughly understand the medical language.

Training is Vital

A patient cannot understand his medical report or record because of its specialized terminology. Coding specialist learns this language through a thorough study program, making it easy for them to comprehend the written word. The next step is for them to translate the report utilizing their professional expertise in the pertinent coding structures. The third-party staff must also be well-informed and trained in comprehending the codes if they review the records and give the proper regulations.

Accuracy of the codes

Experts in medical coding are specialists in a sizable portion of medical data. These professionals convert textual texts into understandable codes. They could struggle to distinguish between two different meanings for the same medical abbreviation if they do not gain practical and in-depth knowledge of the medical regulations.

A coder can carry out his duties effectively and accurately if he thoroughly understands medical documentation standards. After assigning the final codes, accuracy is essential, but a corporation values efficiency. Some medical coders can accurately translate more than 200 records into the required industry-standard code in a single day.

Medical bills and codes are legal documents, just like medical records.

Medical coding specialists offer a transparent and accurate reimbursement process with their professional expertise. Additionally, they ensure that the reports only cover specific services in response to patient health issues.

How Medical Coding Works

The first step in the medical coding process is for the doctor or other healthcare professional to enter their observations and treatments in the patient's medical file. The more thorough this data is, the better the medical coding will reflect the patient's condition and the provided services.

The medical coder reviews the medical record after it has been finished by the doctor, nurse practitioner, or physician assistant. Before the medical coding procedure can be completed, the coder may need to ask the doctor to clarify something if the documentation in the medical record isn't clear. The coder follows a comprehensive set of rules and principles to assign the medical codes that best depict the diagnoses listed in the medical history and the services provided, or operations carried out.

The medical coder frequently uses software to assist with coding a medical record. Software by itself is insufficient, though. To effectively code a medical history, one must also be thoroughly aware of the standards, laws, and ordinances that govern its use and implementation.

After coding the medical record, the medical coder uses the codes to submit a claim to the payer or practice management organization. Health insurers, governmental organizations, and practice management firms examine the medical coding provided with a claim for accuracy. Effective medical coding necessitates close attention to detail and the knowledge of a complicated set of standards.

How to specialize in medical coding: Steps to Becoming a Medical Coder

Medical coding is a fast-expanding industry essential to the healthcare industry's back-end operations. People who work in the healthcare field but would rather not interact directly with patients are an excellent fit for this employment opportunity. Despite this, it calls for an attitude that is focused on the smallest of details as well as a specific set of technical skills.

It's not tough to become a medical coder, but you need some qualifications and an associate's or bachelor's degree in a science-related field. This manual will show you how to select the top medical coding programs, further education opportunities, and the stages of becoming a medical coder.

Step 1: Attend a Postsecondary Institution

Although a postsecondary degree isn't always necessary to work as a medical coder, several certificates demand that candidates have the relevant training. You have several options to choose from, like getting a bachelor's degree, an associate's degree, or completing a certificate program. Your best choice might be to enroll in a medical coding program or school specially made for people who want to work as medical coders.

Step 2: Obtain a basic medical coding license

After completing your school, you can gain specific fundamental qualifications. You are eligible to take the exam for certain credentials even if you do not have any relevant job experience, provided that you have completed the necessary coursework. A couple of examples of credentials are Registered Health Information Technician (RHIT) and Certified Coding Associate (CCA). If you have an associate's degree from a Health Information Management (HIM) school, you are eligible to apply to take the Registered Health Information Technician exam (RHIT).

Step 3: Gain practical experience in the field of medical coding.

You will be able to begin working as a medical coder as soon as you have received the basic certifications that are necessary for the position. There are numerous work environments, including medical offices, hospitals, etc. Many types of medical coding can now be done from home thanks to the growth of remote work.

Step 4: Get Advanced Certifications in Medical Coding in Step Four

After gaining some job experience, you can pursue more advanced degrees to enhance your career. A few years into your career is the optimum time to accomplish certain higher-level credentials.

Step 5: Career Advancement

You will be able to continue working as a medical coder once you have obtained your advanced certification, and you will also have the option to develop your career. One strategy for advancing your career is to take on a leadership job in the form of a manager, consultant, or compliance auditor. You should also consider the possibility of continuing your education to earn a more advanced degree.

Types of medical Code Used

CDT

The American Dental Association owns and maintains CDT codes (ADA). The HCPCS Level II dental section was previously represented by the five-character codes that begin with the letter D.

CPT

The American Medical Association (AMA) owns and maintains the CPT (Current Procedural Terminology) code set, which consists of more than 10,000+ five-character alphanumeric codes defining services rendered to patients by doctors, paraprofessionals, therapists, and others. The CPT® system is used to report the majority of outpatient services. Doctors also use it to document the services they provide to inpatients.

M.S. – DRG

In order for a hospital to get compensated for a patient's stay, the hospital must submit MS-DRGs. The ICD-10-CM and ICD-10-PCS reported codes to form the basis of the MS-DRG. Describe specific patient characteristics, such as the primary diagnosis, particular secondary diagnoses, procedures, sex, and discharge status.

ICD 10

ICD-10-CM contains codes for everything that can harm, ill, or kill you. The 72,000+ code set is made up of codes for ailments, poisons, neoplasms, wounds, their causes, and what people did when the injuries occurred. Codes are "smart codes" that contain up to seven alphanumeric characters and express the patient's complaint in detail.

Procedural Coding System - PCS

Hospitals employ the ICD-10-PCS, a set of more than 78,000 alphanumeric codes, to define surgical procedures in operating rooms, emergency rooms, and other settings.

Level II HCPCS

For the sake of reporting procedures and billing for supplies, Medicare, Medicaid, Blue Cross/Blue Shield, and other providers were the ones who first developed the more than 7,000 alphanumeric codes that make up HCPCS Level II. Still, they are used for various purposes, including academic studies, quality measure tracking, and outpatient surgery billing.

NDC

Every medication packet is tracked and reported using the Federal Drug Administration's (FDA) code. Smart codes with 10–13 alphanumeric characters are used to identify pharmaceuticals prescribed, sold, and utilized by providers, suppliers, and federal agencies.

Modifiers

Hundreds of alphanumeric two-character modifier codes are used in CPT and HCPCS Level II codes to increase clarity. They may denote a patient's status, the body portion on which a service is being rendered, a payment directive, an event that modified the assistance the code refers to, or a quality component.

DRG and APC for MS

MS-DRG and APCs are two federal code sets that are utilized to support payments derived from the systems above. They draw on already-existing code sets but also provide information on the resources needed by the facility to deliver the service.

The Centers for Medicare & Medicaid Services (CMS) are in charge of maintaining an up-to-date version of the Ambulatory Payment Categories (APCs), which are used as a foundation for the Hospital Outpatient Prospective Payment System (HOPPS) (OPPS). This system pays for some of the hospital's outpatient services, including minor surgery and other treatments.

As a medical coder, you are need to be familiar with three distinct forms of coding.

ICD-10-CM

For the purpose of classifying and coding all diagnoses, symptoms, and procedures that are documented in connection with hospital care in the United States, medical professionals and other healthcare professionals use a system known as ICD-10-CM (International Classification of Diseases, Tenth Revision, Clinical Modification). It provides the level of diagnostic specificity and morbidity categorization that are necessary in the United States.

ICD-10-CM, like its predecessor ICD-9-CM, is based on the WHO's International Classification of Diseases, which employs unique alphanumeric codes to designate recognized diseases and other health issues. According to the World Health Organization (WHO), the ICD-10-CM is a tool that helps medical professionals save and retrieve diagnostic data. This tool is utilized by medical coders, health information managers, nurses, and other healthcare workers. ICD records are also utilized in the process of compiling national data on mortality and morbidity.

According to a regulation issued by the United States Department of Health and Human Services, all entities that fall under the purview of the Health Insurance Portability and Accountability Act (HIPAA) are required to make use of the ICD-10-CM code set (HHS).

ICD-10-CM codes and their significance

The significance of ICD-10-CM codes lies in the fact that they are more specific than ICD-10 codes and may provide extra information indicating the severity of a patient's ailment.

CPT

Most medical operations in a doctor's office are documented using Current Procedure Terminology, or CPT, codes. This code set is published by the American Medical Association, which is also responsible for its maintenance (AMA). The AMA has copyright protection for these codes, which are updated yearly.

CPT codes are a three-category system of five-digit numerical codes. The first category, the six ranges, is the most frequently utilized. These ranges relate to six critical medical specialties: medicine, pathology, anesthesia, surgery, radiology, and evaluation and management.

The second group of CPT codes relates to performance evaluation and, occasionally, the findings of radiological or laboratory tests. These hyphenated, five-digit alphanumeric codes are frequently appended to the end of Category I CPT codes.

Category II codes are optional; they cannot replace Category I codes. These codes are helpful for other doctors and healthcare providers, and the AMA hopes that Category II codes will lessen the administrative burden on doctors' offices by giving them access to more and better data about the effectiveness of healthcare providers and facilities.

Emerging medical technology is categorized under the third CPT code category.

Though the first will be more frequent, as a coder, you'll spend most of your time working on the first two groups.

In addition, CPT codes can have addenda that enhance the code's specificity and ensure that it is entered correctly. The American Medical Association (AMA) developed a series of CPT modifiers due to the fact that many medical treatments require a higher acceptable degree of data than what is provided by the fundamental Category I CPT code. The Category I CPT code is followed by one of these two-digit numeric or alphanumeric codes. CPT modifiers give the procedure code valuable further information. For instance, a CPT modifier can be used to specify which side of the patient's body a procedure would be performed.

HCPCS

When submitting claims for healthcare to Medicare or any other health insurer, medical providers are required to utilize the Healthcare Common Procedure Coding System (HCPCS), which is a standardized code system. This ensures that the claims are uniform and organized. HCPCS Level I and Level II are two medical code sets.

For the purpose of filing medical claims to payers, HCPCS Level I is utilized. These claims might be for procedures and services rendered by physicians, non-physicians, hospitals, labs, and outpatient facilities. It includes all of the codes that make up the Current Procedural Terminology (CPT®) set.

The HCPCS Level II national procedure code set is utilized by healthcare professionals, providers, and suppliers of medical equipment when filing claims to health plans for medical devices, supplies, medications, transportation services, and other products and services.

HCPCS Level II codes are often mentioned when medical coders and billers discuss HCPCS codes. They genuinely mean HCPCS Level I when they speak of CPT® coding.

In a manner analogous to that of CPT codes, each HCPCS code need to be accompanied with a diagnostic code that lends support to the medical procedure. It is the job of the coders to ensure that every outpatient operation stated in the medical report makes sense in light of the given diagnosis, usually indicated by an ICD code.

Some Medical Coding Models

What Is SNOMED CT?

SNOMED CT, which stands for Systematized Nomenclature of Medicine - Clinical Terms, is a dictionary of standardized clinical terms that is available in multiple languages. This makes it simpler for medical professionals to communicate important information with one another. It is regarded as the world's most complete vocabulary of clinical terminology.

Symptoms, signs, diagnoses, treatments, clinical findings, and body structures are some of the terms whose definitions are recorded in SNOMED CT. These terms are frequently used in the context of healthcare. In addition to this, its database has the ability to differentiate between different etiologies, drugs, samples, and pieces of medical equipment.

This system currently serves as the basis for the development of interoperable software that is relevant to health, and it is at the center of the information systems that are used to keep electronic medical records.

How does SNOMED CT work?

Each SNOMED CT component and derivative type is related to and represented in a specific fashion according to the SNOMED CT logical model. In SNOMED CT, concepts, descriptions, and relationships are the three main components. Our approach outlines the management of the components in an implementation scenario to accommodate various primary and secondary purposes.

Why Snomed, CT?

Individual patients, physicians, and populations all gain from SNOMED CT-based clinical information, which also helps evidence-based therapy. SNOMED CT can represent pertinent clinical information wholly and consistently as a crucial component of electronic health information when used in software programs for Electronic Health Records.

Rules have defined SNOMED CT as the U.S. national standard for new health information exchange transactions and additional types of information in EHRs. SNOMED CT has been adopted as the standard for specific data items in worldwide genetic information resources such as the Genetic Testing Registry and the database of clinically significant human variants being developed at the NIH. Both of these resources are examples of worldwide genetic information resources. Additionally, more and more clinical research investigations are using it.

What Is LOINC?

A centralized database called LOINC (Logical Observation Identifiers Names and Codes) facilitates the exchange and collection of clinical results, including lab tests, clinical observations, and patient outcomes related to measurements. Healthcare administration and laboratory testing equipment also use it.

Both laboratory competence and research are made easier by LOINC's provision of a common vocabulary for describing the various results obtained. The Regenstrief Institute, Inc. was the organization responsible for the creation, maintenance, and operation of the LOINC database.

Why is LOINC used?

To make the communication of laboratory findings between healthcare organizations easier, LOINC was created in 1994. Laboratory test codes were distinct from one another before it was created, and data could not be sent and received across healthcare providers.

How is LOINC maintained?

The Regenstrief Institute, a nonprofit organization based in Indiana that does healthcare research, developed and maintained LOINC. In June and December, LOINC updates are made available twice a year.

What do LOINC codes look like?

There are six sections to LOINC code descriptions, each of which has a distinct meaning. They are alphanumeric and, in contrast to other code sets, have a structure that is more like a phrase.

There is a potential for employment as a "Remote Medical Coder."

The future of medical coding seems promising due to the fact that individuals in the United States are living longer and there are more people overall. Medical billing and coding are complementary tasks that are a staple of medical office work. Coders produce precise patient data that can be used in the future and are used by the billing department to make statements. These documents are sent to insurance providers and, ultimately, patients.

Medical coders use internationally standardized alphanumeric coding. It is made up of the languages that are used for the Current Procedural Terminology (CPT) and the International Classification of Diseases (ICD). They translate doctors' memoranda and reports into these two coding schemes for use by patients, insurance providers, and other third parties for billing.

Pay for Remote Medical Coding Jobs

It is typical to locate remote coding jobs that pay hourly, even if some businesses that hire medical coders online pay by the chart. Remote medical coding employment typically spends between $28 and $35 per hour.

The amount you make as a medical coder depends on your experience, certifications, and the type of coding you do. For example, jobs in inpatient medical coding typically pay more than outpatient medical coding jobs.

Experience Required

Most remote medical coding job openings require at least a year of prior coding experience. This suggests that if you are just starting out in the field of medical coding, the first job you get will most likely be a local one rather than a remote one. If you don't have much coding knowledge, it would be worthwhile to perform some web study to find out more about 99213. Above all, learning more about medical coding can never be started too late. There will always be possibilities to learn about the nuances of natural language processing in healthcare and investigate cutting-edge healthcare software further, even if there are positions you want to apply for right now.

How to Get a Job Coding Medical Records From Home

It is wise to deal with a medical staffing agency to get your next remote medical coding job because the firm will only present you with openings from trustworthy employers and will be actively working on your behalf as they normally get paid after placing an employee. The most excellent place to start is with your fellow medical coders if you decide to look for a remote medical coding job on your own. They probably have contacts or have learned about different employers from other programmers.

Work Schedule and Accountability

Working remotely as a medical coder might include a wide range of hours. You may be able to work any hours you like as long as you meet the minimum requirements each day or each week for some coding jobs. Like most in-person occupations, other medical coding positions will have a predetermined schedule you must adhere to. It's important to discuss availability during the hiring process before accepting a job offer. Be aware that minor coding roles typically have very high production accountability. The employer will probably conduct a thorough audit of your accuracy and productivity, and they want you to always adhere to their timetable standards.

Preparation for a Career in Medical Coding That Can Be Carried Out From Home

Ensure you understand how you will be trained to work within the system before accepting a position. Using their method without assistance is impossible, in my opinion. When you work remotely as a coder, you could have odd hours, which means that the people who can assist you if you run into trouble might not be accessible when you need them. As a result, you should have as many on-demand resources as possible to assist you in navigating the employer's system. Screenshots, a digital manual that details their system, on-demand training videos, and pre-recorded training are some examples of tools you should have on hand.

Equipment and Software Needed

Discover what they anticipate having in your home office before accepting a remote medical coding job. Some employers will give you a computer, while others will demand you bring your own. You must learn the system requirements to operate the software used by your workplace if you are needed to use a personal computer. Find out if their system is cloud-based or requires you to install their software on your P.C. Find out whether their I.T. staff will help you with the installation if you need to put their software on your P.C.

Online Training for Medical Coding Positions

Before agreeing to work remotely in medical coding, it is important to find out whether or not the company will pay for your continuing education units (CEUs) and whether or not you will be compensated for the time it will take you to complete the CEUs.

AHIMA and AAPC certification options.

Medical coders are crucial parts of the healthcare team because, without correct medical coding, hospitals, doctors, and patients might not receive the full insurance reimbursement.

The choice of which coding certification is best for you will need to be made if you're considering becoming a medical coder. To learn more about medical coding and your certification possibilities, keep reading.

What Are the Benefits of Getting Certified?

Although certification is not necessary, there are many significant advantages to doing so.

- greater pay
- improved employability
- career development
- personal development
- professional relationships
- more flexibility in the workplace
- increased options for education

Working remotely from home is possible with several medical coding certificates that assess your proficiency with one of three code sets and one of three levels of coding.

Certificates in medical coding

There are numerous certificates in medical coding, including:

1. Certified Professional Coder (CPC)
2. Certified Outpatient Coding (COC)
3. Certified Inpatient Coder (CIC)
4. Certified Coding Specialist (CCS)
5. Certified Medical Coder (CMC)

Let's look at each of them separately to help you better understand how the certifications differ from one another.

Certified Professional Coder (CPC)

The Certified Professional Coder is a credential recognized by the American Academy of Professional Coders (CPC).

Who Does the Cpc Work For?

Those aspiring to careers as medical coders in outpatient settings like clinics and doctors' offices should aim for the CPC. The CPC increases the earning potential by more than $25,000 over other annual incomes, according to the AAPC. And it's the most well-known credential for medical coders.

Exam CPC

The current COVID-19 outbreak has forced the CPC exam to be made available online in addition to the traditional in-person format. The cost is between $299 and $399, depending on whether you choose to enroll in person or online.

Certified Outpatient Coding (COC)

The American Academy of Professional Coders has accredited the COC certification (formerly the CPC-H), which shows a high degree of coding proficiency, particularly in hospital groups, ambulatory surgery facilities, and hospital billing and coding departments.

For Whom Is The Coc Suitable?

For coders who work in hospitals, there is a COC certification.

Exam COC

There are 150 multiple-choice questions in the COC exam. It will take you approximately 5 hours and 40 minutes to finish the exam. The exam costs $399 ($325 for AAPC students) and comes with one free retake.

Certified Inpatient Coder (CIC)

The only certification exclusively for inpatient hospital/facility coding is the Certified Inpatient Coder (CIC), recognized by the American Academy of Professional Coders.

For Whom Is The Cic Suitable?

As we previously stated, this certification is intended for individuals working in inpatient hospitals or facilities and calls for a thorough understanding of inpatient codes, medical processes, and inpatient procedures. It necessitates that the ICD-10-PCS procedure and ICD-10-CM diagnosis codes be utilized correctly when coding and paying insurance companies for inpatient hospital care.

Exam CIC

There are 60 multiple-choice questions and ten inpatient cases on the CIC certification test. It will take you approximately 5 hours and 40 minutes to finish the exam. For $399 (or $325 for AAPC students), you get one free trial.

Certified Coding Specialist (CCS)

The Certified Coding Specialist (CCS) certification, accredited by the American Health Information Management Association (AHIMA), is used to code medical data used by hospitals and other healthcare facilities to obtain payment from insurance providers or government programs like Medicare and Medicaid.

For Whom Are The Ccs Suitable?

Medical coders with competence in coding inpatient and outpatient data are eligible for the Certified Coding Specialist (CCS) certification.

Exam CCS

A multiple-choice component and a medical scenario section make up the exam. The test has a four-hour time limit. And to pass, you must receive a grade of at least 300.

Certified Medical Coder (CMC)

The Practice Management Institute offers the Certified Medical Coder (CMC) certification, regarded as one of the most widespread and well-liked medical coding credentials (PMI).

For Whom Is The Cmc Suitable?

Despite its popularity, this certification's testing format makes it more challenging than exams for other medical coding certifications. Only medical coders working in an outpatient setting are eligible for the CMC certification.

Exam CMC

The PMI offers a review course to aid in exam preparation due to the difficulty of the exam. Although not required, it is strongly advised for success.

The PMI website lists several advantages to acquiring a CMC, including,

A CMC safeguards the practice's financial stability by reducing claim rejections, enhancing billing accuracy, and ensuring compliance with current regulations.

A CMC does not rely on web searches, coding cheat sheets, or EHR presets for coding assignments, which might result in reoccurring issues and lead to an audit.

A CMC can develop into supervisory and chart auditing jobs because they can confidently engage with doctors, third-party payers, patients, and business partners.

How to use codes after a diagnosis

To run a successful billing business, medical billing businesses and healthcare providers must thoroughly understand CMS 1500 & UB-04 forms. The National Uniform Claim Committee is responsible for creating and updating these forms (NUCC). CMS 1500 & UB-04, which are explicitly used for revenue payments, vary.

Knowing the form to submit a claim on is crucial for obtaining the proper compensation. The most typical claim forms sent to insurance companies are CMS-1500 & UB-04. Both have their unique standards, although they are both extremely often utilized, making the medical billing process work smoothly.

Let's delve further into the UB-04 and CMS 1500 forms.

I need to know about the UB-04 and CMS 1500 forms.

CMS 1500:

- The National Uniform Claim Committee, which is also known as NUCC, is responsible for the creation of this form, which is also known as the 1500 or HCFA. The purpose of this form was to serve as the standard for healthcare providers, including individual physicians, nurses, and other medical practices.

- When submitting claims to Medicare and regional carriers for durable medical equipment, non-institutional providers who are not subject to the Administrative Simplification Compliance Act's mandate that all claims be submitted electronically must use the CMS-1500 standard claim form. Further, it is used for billing purposes by a number of state agencies that participate in Medicaid.The CMS 1500 form is used to generate bills for medical services provided by healthcare professionals in settings such as hospitals and ambulatory surgical centers.

- Even if the same provider is providing the services, the facility will not be billed using this form even though it was provided by that provider.

- Both the CMS 1500 and the UB-04 forms have their own unique methods for billing patients for the procedures or services that medical professionals render.

- The procedure for making a claim will not be completed until these two forms have been submitted.

UB-04:

- The UB-04 form was introduced in 2005 as a direct replacement for the UB-92 form. This form has been standardized for usage since more than 15 years ago, and it is mostly utilized by hospitals, ambulatory surgery centers, nursing homes, and other institutions for both the physical and emotional health of patients.
- The fact that the UB-04 can either be submitted on paper or in an electronic format is the form's defining characteristic.
- Insurance firms will continue to employ the filing procedures they have in place, whether it is to receive these documents on paper or online. There are several states that cannot process these forms. On this point, they differ from one another.
- The one and only time that this does not apply is when hospitals or other medical facilities are billing Medicare. When submitting a claim, you must use the CMS 1500 form because Medicare is the only payer that accepts it.
- The term "Uniform Billing," abbreviated as "UB" in UB-04, is also referred to as "CMS 1450." The process of submitting a claim has been standardized and made more efficient by the creation of the UB-04 form by the Centers for Medicare and Medicaid Services.

Explain how to prepare to make an error-free claim

The complications of medical billing and coding are numerous. Specifically, the long list of codes can stump even the most competent and well-organized billing personnel. The financial health of your practice might suffer from even minor errors.

Because of this, our medical billing experts have compiled the top 10 techniques to prevent errors and mistakes:

Use the most recent coding guide

Never refer to an out-of-date code manual. To stay current with standards, you should regularly update your guides and coding techniques by attending seminars. You and your patients should experience relief due to a more streamlined billing procedure for your claims.

Emphasize cross-border services

X-rays, shots, pills, and other treatments are considered bilateral services. Coders must openly emphasize the services to make users aware of their inclusion. In remote work, the emphasis is essential to alert the billers in case the doctor misses it.

Keep track of the advantages offered.

If you can check the benefits offered at their source beforehand, you can avoid making many mistakes. You can use any recently entered information with no problem if it's an old patient. Errors may occur if the patient's details, such as the insurance company, policy limit, or terms of service, change. Therefore, it's crucial to always double-check the information for both new and existing patients. Communicate with the insurer any authorizations already in place, those that have been sent, co-payment alternatives, healthcare benefits, and the duration of coverage. Verifying every piece of information properly will be essential to preventing billing mistakes.

Don't upgrade

Never report a minor procedure as a major one since the insurer could have to compensate the healthcare provider at a higher rate. Try to avoid upcoding, whether done intentionally or not, if you want to prevent future compliance and legal problems. As a result, always provide proper codes to prevent claims rejection and legal disputes. If there is an upcoding issue, your practice could be severely penalized.

Check for Any Wrong Information or Typographical Errors

The slightest and most elementary errors in patient information can ultimately result in the rejection of a claim. A simple mistake can ruin the billing procedure with a patient's name, birthday, or gender. Incorrect policy and group numbers for claims or prior authorizations are also covered.

Select the Best EHR System

Your claim will be rejected if the written prescription is difficult to understand. Choosing the appropriate EHR for your practice will help you cut down on errors. Your team must be instructed to ask inquiries and verify any ambiguous coding or services provided. Additionally, you can link your EHR and automated billing systems. To guarantee a seamless billing process, the personnel will need rigorous training.

Give complete information

Payment denial or delay will result from providing incomplete data. The processing of claims may be impacted by failing to include a fourth and fifth digit or by failing to associate a diagnosis code with a Current Procedural Terminology (CPT) Healthcare Common Procedure Coding System (HCPCS) code. Although human error is the primary culprit, incorrect diagnosis data may also be to blame.

Raise Coding QA Standards

Ensure that the procedure codes and diagnoses are accurate for a successful reimbursement of medical claims. The following things could render claims invalid:

- The insurance company makes false assumptions
- Wrong codes
- No need for treatments is medical
- An action is taken without permission.

Refrain from billing twice

To minimize difficulties from double billing, always conduct audits. The provision of procedure invoices for canceled or rescheduled procedures increases the possibility of claim denials, making it one of the prevalent blunders. But implementing chart audits will stop the spread of these mistakes.

Name your Coding

Since some ICD-10 codes require the last two numbers to be precise to prevent a denial, it is the coder's responsibility to take precautions to ensure that each code is correct. When coders are unsure about whether a diagnosis has been accurately coded or not, it is convenient to consult the codebook.

How Difficult Is It, Really, to Learn Medical Coding?

You may be curious about the difficulty of medical coding training if you're thinking about enrolling. The answer? You must be committed and have a strong work ethic in addition to your selected program.

Though it can be incredibly lucrative, the profession of medical coding is challenging. How to get the most out of medical coding training will be covered in this blog post, along with what to anticipate. We'll also debunk a few myths regarding medical coding that might prevent you from pursuing this profession!

Medical coding refers to the practice of assigning numeric identifiers to medical concepts including diagnosis, procedures, and treatments. These codes are employed to track patient health data and charge insurance companies.

Who requires a medical coder?

Medical coders provide accurate billing and payment information to healthcare providers. In fact, without medical coders, many healthcare companies could not run!

How is training in medical coding conducted?

Medical coders can work without a degree in medicine and a specific license, but they still need to be well-versed in medical language and anatomy.

Understanding the rules governing patient privacy is necessary for medical coding, which requires in-depth knowledge of medical vocabulary and processes (HIPAA). Coders in this field need to be able to take raw patient data and turn it into billable codes using specialized software.

What sort of instruction do I require?

Medical coding training programs come in various formats, including certificate, associate, and bachelor degrees. Your degree of experience and professional ambitions will determine the kind of program you enroll in.

Usually lasting 12 months or less, certificate programs concentrate on teaching the fundamentals of medical coding.

Associate's degrees last a little longer (18 months on average) and include a more thorough introduction to medical coding.

Bachelor's degrees normally take four years to finish and entail coursework in medical coding and billing.

How hard is it?

While it's true that medical coding classes might be difficult, it's important to keep in mind that the knowledge you gain will be useful in your future career. If you are dedicated and willing to put in the effort, you will be successful in this line of work.

Exams for certification are available from the American Academy of Professional Coders (AAPC), which evaluates your coding knowledge and skills. You must succeed on an AAPC exam to be certified.

So, how challenging is learning medical coding? Your medical coding qualification may be relevant. The medical coding training course you select will impact how difficult and time-consuming the examinations are.

Explain how to handle contractual disputes and appeals

What Is a Provider Dispute?

A formal notification to Health Net from the non-participating provider that:

- Challenges, appeals, or demands reconsideration of a claim that has been rejected, changed, or contested (including a bundled collection of related claims).
- examines a request for repayment for an excessive claim payment
- seeks to resolve a billing disagreement or another contractual conflict

Time Limit for Provider Disputes

As specified below, Health Net accepts provider complaints lodged within 365 days after receiving Health Net's decision (for instance, Health Net's Remittance Advice (RA) indicating a claim was denied or amended). A dispute about the claim must be lodged within 365 days after the statutory deadline for Health Net to contest or deny the claim has passed if the provider does not receive a claim determination from Health Net.

Disputes from Providers to Be Submitted

In order to file a provider disagreement, a provider is required to fill out a Provider Dispute Resolution Request form.

The name, ID number, contact information, phone number, and the same claim number assigned to the provider must all be included in the provider dispute. If the dispute pertains to a claim or a request for reimbursement of an overpayment of a claim, there are several different pieces of information that are required. A clear identification of the disputed item, the date of service, and a clear justification of why the provider thinks the payment amount, a request for further information, a request for the return of an overpayment, or another action is incorrect are examples of these pieces of information.

A thorough discussion of the topic and the foundation for the provider's stance if the disagreement is unrelated to a claim.

When a disagreement with a provider is presented on behalf of a member, the member appeal mechanism handles the dispute. A provider is deemed to support a member with their member appeal when they file a dispute on the member's behalf.

If it is a member-related problem, the dispute must include the member's name, ID number, a clear explanation of the disputed item, the date of service, the billed and paid amounts, and the provider's position.

All provider disputes and supporting documentation must be sent to the following:

Suppose the provider dispute does not contain the essential components of a submission. In that case, as described above, it is sent back to the provider with a written statement asking for the required information to settle the issue. Within the time limit for dispute submissions, the provider must resubmit a modified dispute with the missing data. The amended argument must have all the data needed to resolve the dispute.

As part of the claims adjudication process, Health Net does not ask providers to resubmit claim data or supporting materials unless the provider has already received the data back from Health Net.

The fact that a provider has used the provider dispute process does not result in Health Net engaging in discrimination or retaliation against that provider.

Recognizing Provider Disputes

Within the first 15 business days after receipt, Health Net will acknowledge receipt of each provider dispute, regardless of whether or not the dispute is resolved.

Resolution period

When Health Net receives a disagreement from a provider, it addresses the issue as quickly as possible—within 45 business days—and then sends the provider a written decision with an explanation of its reasoning.

Paid in the past

If the disagreement between the provider and Health Net concerns a claim, and the provider prevails, Health Net will pay any money that is still owed to the provider, including any applicable interest or penalties, within five business days of the decision. After the day that the claim should have been handled, interest and penalties, if there are any, will begin to accumulate on the next day.

Costs of Dispute Resolution

The processing of a provider dispute is free of charge for the provider. However, Health Net is not obligated to pay the provider back for any expenses paid during the procedure.

Chapter 4: Medical Billing

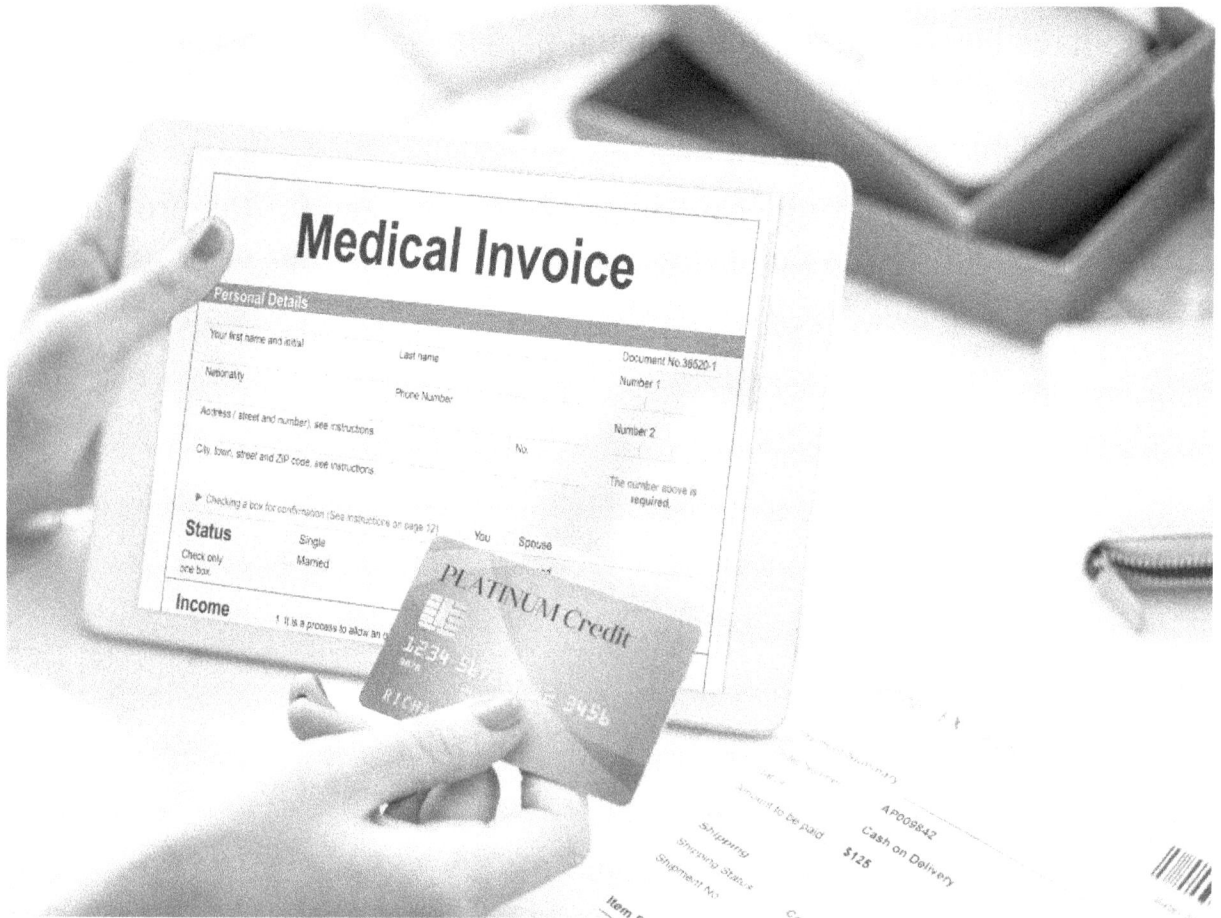

Explain how to negotiate medical bills and laboratory fees

If you've ever had a high-priced medical bill, you might not have thought about negotiating the price. Instead, you could have had to make difficult life decisions to figure out how to make the payments or consider borrowing money. Knowing what you require and who to contact to negotiate your bill may result in a cheaper account and less worry for you.

The high cost of essential medical services and treatments can result in further financial strain or complete for the goal of care.

Verify the bill for mistakes.

This can be challenging because medical bills employ specific terminology, but if you know where to look, you can tell if your account is accurate.

Almost all processes are designed to make it easier for insurance companies to collect payments. You can conduct an online search to learn what the medical codes on your bills mean. Compare the definitions of the procedures to the ones you've had done so that you may find out if you are being charged for the treatment that you've had.

Some mistakes are surprisingly frequent:

- There is a chance that the codes will not match your diagnosis. If the codes don't match, your insurance, if you have one, will probably refuse to cover any portion of this claim.
- Upcoding is when you receive a bill for a procedure that isn't the one you had, even if it may be comparable and generally costs more.
- Duplicate billing, or several billings for the same treatment, is one example of a mistake.
- Additionally, services that ought to have been invoiced under a single umbrella diagnosis or code are separated in a process known as unbundling, which frequently results in higher costs.

Speak with a Billing Department or Administrator

Start the negotiation process by filing a letter of settlement request. If you want to avoid a payment plan, here is a beautiful place to start when outlining the details you have discovered and the sum you are willing to pay. Make sure that your request may be considered both reasonable and respectful. You will have a better chance of getting your settlement offer accepted by the medical offices if you can pay your requested amount in full.

Pan predicts that you'll need to be persistent. Ask how to file a settlement letter and how long it usually takes to analyze by calling the billing department. You need to make sure that they have got your letter by checking in with them during the subsequent few days. You can frequently find this phone number right there on your statement, so keep it close at hand.

Additionally, administrators may provide interest-free payment arrangements. Ask the hospital what discounts they offer or if you are eligible for a financial aid program or charity care if you are interested in a payment plan. Although many for-profit hospitals also provide these services, all nonprofit hospitals are legally mandated to do so. Having your most current tax return on hand may help your case because you might be eligible for a lower cost based on your income.

Always keep a record of what was said, when it happened, and who you spoke with during these calls. Your credit may benefit from having supporting documentation for future usage. It is crucial to have written confirmation of this agreement regarding the new bill, such as a settlement letter.

Do your research.

Find out how much surgery will cost before undergoing it. Request from your physician the actual operation name or, if possible, the billing code or Current Procedural Terminology (CPT). You also need to be aware of the specifics and deductibles of your insurance coverage. It will be much simpler to bargain for medical costs if you are prepared with this information. Even better, you always have the option of using a firm that can negotiate your medical payments for you!

Get an itemized bill

McClanahan advised requesting an itemized bill so you could check it and confirm the charges were accurate.

Errors might include erroneous patient, provider, or insurance information, incorrect procedure codes, and duplicate billing, among other things.

For instance, the medical billing error detection company Medliminal often discovers that 25% of the charges on the evaluated bills are not billable.

How the insurance process works

What is Medical Insurance Billing?

Medical insurance billing refers to the process of making a claim and following up on it in order to get reimbursement for services given by a healthcare practitioner. Medical billers in healthcare facilities follow up on claims made in response to medical services to get payment.

The Method of Medical Billing

The reality that each insurance company, each operation, and each provider will impact the process and the financial outcome is at the core of the complexity associated with the medical billing process.

The use of optimal medical billing practices by industry professionals is essential to ensure that they are operating effectively and efficiently. This entails taking advantage of folks who are skilled and committed to producing high-quality work for the supplier.

- Numerous broad factors can change how the charging process operates.
- An overview of a medical billing workflow can be found here.

Patient Registration

The first stage on any flow chart depicting the billing process for medical services is patient registration. In this section, fundamental biographical information about a patient is gathered, such as their name, birthday, and the primary purpose of their visit. Medical billers are responsible for gathering and verifying patient insurance information, including the patient's policy number and the insurance provider's name. Billers in the medical industry are responsible for collecting and verifying insurance information, including the patient's policy number and the name of the insurance provider.

Verify the patient's insurance.

Verifying insurance can be relatively simple. After collecting the patient's insurance information, you should get in touch with the insurer to get the details confirmed.

In most cases, the insurance card of a patient will have a contact number that may be dialed in order to verify the information on the card. When you talk to a representative from the insurance company, make sure to ask them about the patient's coverage and the benefits to which they are entitled. In order to determine how much to charge the patient, you should inquire about their copays and deductibles.

Superbill Creation

The patient will be required to fill out paperwork for their file upon check-in, or if it's a return visit, to verify or amend information already on file. Along with taking identification and any necessary co-payments, you will be needed to present an insurance card that is currently active. Following the patient's departure, the medical records from the visit are translated by a medical coder into diagnostic and procedural codes. The information gathered until that point might then be combined to create an account known as a "superbill." It will include details about the clinician and provider, the patient's demographics and medical history, the procedures and services provided, as well as the diagnosis and procedure codes that are applicable.

In order to properly code medical procedures, you need to take notes either while the patient is being seen or immediately afterwards. List your services, diagnosis, treatments, and medications in detail. It is highly recommended that you store this information within your electronic medical record system.

Why Hospitals are Automating Billing

The billing and receivables workforce is expensive for many providers and is sometimes to blame for inaccurate coding and billing, which results in delayed revenue. The medical sector's transition to automated billing reduces mistakes, time, and expense.

"All too frequently, insurance companies find tactics to evade or postpone payment for legitimate medical claims," we've said. One approach to ensure that insurance companies looking to undermine providers have nowhere to stand is to use the most recent technologies.

Utilizing technology makes it more challenging to attribute problems to a breakdown in clear communication.

Billing Health Insurance

Insurance firms have a reputation for processing claims slowly or erroneously. Knowing how the process operates will help everyone avoid being caught off guard when something goes wrong and ensure that patients and providers receive what they should.

In the past, health insurance providers have avoided being honest. Denied claims are an inevitable part of the system, whether due to sneaky tactics where they try to escape liability or something more obvious like an unfulfilled deductible. Understanding how they function is absolutely necessary in order to make the process as simple and uncomplicated as it can possibly be.

Do I ever have to submit an insurance claim on my own, or does the medical facility handle that?

- Usually, you won't need to submit a claim by hand.
- The majority of healthcare professionals handle this procedure. However, if you ever need to submit an insurance claim on your own, follow these guidelines to ensure a smooth claim processing process:
- Write legibly and concisely.
- It is in your best interest to turn in your documentation as quickly as possible and well before the deadline.
- If necessary, include preapproval.
- Include all necessary details

- Include procedure codes, which you can obtain from your doctor's office.
- Please make use of the claim form that was provided by your benefits plan.
- Make sure your specific plan covers the services you received.
- The claim procedure is the same, except you must submit the documentation. However, you might need to pay your doctor up front and wait for your health insurance to reimburse you.

Does my choice of health insurance plan impact how insurance claims are processed?

You can anticipate that your claims procedure will operate consistently across insurance providers. However, if you must pay in advance and file your claim after receiving care, you might have to wait for your health insurance provider to repay you.

To completely comprehend how they handle payment and claim processing, speak with your health insurance provider and organization.

Which categories of payers have an impact on the process of reimbursement?

Healthcare practitioners are paid by insurance, or the government pays through a payment system. After you have received medical care, the provider will send the bills for those charges to the person who is responsible for paying them.

The amount that will be billed to you is based on the cost of the treatment itself as well as the predetermined amount that Medicare or your health insurance provider has opted to pay for that service. To determine how much Medicare will pay for a procedure, look it up using the standard procedural technology (CPT) code.

With providers and hospitals, private insurance firms set their payment rates.

People whose insurance doesn't reimburse them enough are often turned away from hospitals and other medical providers, unless the situation is life-threatening.

Co-Pay and Co-Insurance

Your health insurance policy's coverage contract should make it abundantly apparent whether or not you will be required to pay a co-payment or a co-insurance premium for the medical services you get.

Paying the Balance

Imagine that the provider of your healthcare services agrees to take your insurance as payment for the services they deliver. In that case, it indicates that your payer has already made payment and that there will be no additional cost to you beyond your co-pay and co-insurance.

Balance billing is the practice of invoicing you for more money than initially agreed upon without informing you beforehand. In most cases, balance billing is prohibited.

Your Share of the Cost for Additional Services

You might have to pay out-of-pocket for procedures and services not covered by your insurance, even if you have health insurance. You are responsible for this cost, which is distinct from balance billing.

In particular, if they insist you have a choice for the treatment within your network, your insurer may refuse to pay for your care if you decide to go outside your network. In some circumstances, your provider can charge you more than your insurance covers.

Concierge care, in which you enter a contract with a medical facility or practice to receive special attention, typically entails high expenditures not paid for by your health insurance.

Self Pay

Your healthcare practitioner must tell you the cost of services if you are paying for your medical treatment out of pocket. However, be aware that some expenditures can be unforeseen.

For instance, if you have a diagnostic procedure, you could develop a reaction to the contrast medium. Treating your allergic reaction may be required as a result of this. If you were unaware of the allergy before your test, it was impossible to budget for the cost of that service.

Health Reimbursement Arrangement (HRA)

There are employers in the United States who provide their staff members health reimbursement plans (HRAs). They pay for the employees' out-of-pocket medical costs. They must be included in a group health insurance plan and are not given as the only benefit.

An HRA is paid for by the employer, who also benefits financially because the employee is not subject to income tax on the money.

If your health plan has a high deductible, an HRA may be advantageous as it will allow you to get reimbursement for medical costs before you hit the deductible limit.

Understanding Your Medical Bills

Depending on the number of services that you have obtained, a medical bill could either appear simple or quite complicated to you. Generally, you ought to see the name of the service, its total cost, and your own cost. Finding these items in the bill, however, can take some time.

Fee-for-service (FFS), capitation, and bundled payments/episode-based payments have traditionally been the three most common primary forms of payment utilized in the healthcare sector. Below is a description of different reimbursement approaches' structures and any possible unintended outcomes.

Fee for Service (FFS)

A physician's income under the FFS reimbursement model is contingent on the treatments that they provide. The particular "services" that a patient receives would each have their own unique code and associated cost. For instance, different regulations and expenses are associated with a 15-minute clinic visit, a tetanus shot, a urinalysis, and a basic metabolic profile.

Additionally, the healthcare professional's payment for a particular service depends on the patient's insurance. When working with Medicare or Medicaid, the Centers for Medicare and Medicaid Services is responsible for determining the pricing on a per-code basis (CMS).

The cost of commercial (or private) insurance is sometimes expressed as a percentage of the cost of Medicare. Medicaid has the most affordable rates, followed by Medicare, and then commercial insurance comes in last. To put it another way, a doctor might be paid three times as much to treat a patient with private insurance as they would treat one with Medicaid.

Since a provider's primary method to raise their revenue is by performing more services, FFS reimbursement approaches are often known as "volume-based" reimbursement. A clinician must demonstrate that the patient's current diagnoses justify the operations they do to receive payment. Here, there is a potential for an incentive mismatch since doctors may feel justified in providing additional services (and earning more money as a result) even if the patient may not require or benefit from them.

Capitation

In its most basic form, capitation is a payment made to a provider to cover all services for a given population over an extended period. For instance, a doctor's practice with 100 patients would receive $25 per month to cover all expenses related to those patients for the month. Although one patient may use $0 in services and another may use $5,000, the provider will still receive $25. The payment amount has no direct relationship to the number of services rendered.

Capitation takes many distinct shapes. While some capitation payments cover professional charges (such as the cost of seeing a primary care physician or specialist), others reimburse all patient expenses (hospital inpatient, outpatient, and pharmacy).

To make the remuneration more "fair," numerous alterations can be made to the capitation payment. For instance, it would not be fair for a doctor to earn the same $25 per patient that a doctor who exclusively treats young adults would receive because Medicare patients are typically older and sicker. Doctors would be motivated to treat younger, exclusively healthier patients in this environment.

The capitation payment may be adjusted depending on various variables, including the patient's age and gender, location (service fees may vary by zip code), and state of health (chronic conditions). However, it can be difficult to properly and effectively adjust capitation payments for altering health status. Most of the time, the reimbursement for the sickest patients is insufficient to pay all their expenses.

Capitation (or fixed) reimbursement models, as opposed to volume-based reimbursement structures, permit physicians to raise revenue by accepting more patients. Suppose a doctor receives $X per patient regardless of his services. Because of this, his motive is to bring in as many patients as possible, which frequently results in a reduction in the quality of therapy as well as the amount of time spent with each individual patient.

One type of fixed remuneration is the salary paid to medical professionals. Although there is no motivation for doctors to deliver as many services or to see as many patients as possible when they are paid salaries, there is still a gap between the payment received (fixed wage) and the services rendered. Providers servicing older/sicker populations will receive the same compensation for performing more work, similar to the capitation scenario mentioned above. In addition, how should pay be adjusted from one year to the next if there is a significant shift in either the number of patients served or the quality of the services provided?

Bundled Payments / Episode-Based Payments

The funding of health care providers is based on anticipated expenses for clinically defined episodes of care and is known as a bundled or episode-based payment. These episodes deal with various medical issues, such as maternity care, hip replacements, cancer, and organ transplants. As a result, even though some individual surgeries would cost more and some will cost less, a provider would get compensated $10,000 for every hip replacement he performs, for instance, if the projected cost of an easy hip replacement is $10,000.

A capitation plan combined with a fee-for-service reimbursement model is an example of what is known as bundled payments. Only for what is anticipated to be necessary, providers get paid for all of the different specific procedures that are necessary as part of the overall episode of care. A provider will receive less money for the care episode if their circumstance is more severe than what was taken into account while pricing the episode. As with capitation, it is crucial to consider different episode severity levels in pricing. The bundled payment system encourages efficient care since providers can raise their revenue by cutting costs if the pricing accurately reflects the severity.

The acceptance of bundled payments has increased since the ACA's adoption. They have been applied as a tactic to lower medical expenses by improving the quality of services. Medicare and private insurers have expressed interest in bundled payments to cut costs. Effectively utilizing this reimbursement mechanism is difficult, though. It is challenging to determine suitable projected expenses per episode, especially for illnesses like cancer that have an extensive range in cost and severity. It can be tricky to calculate the cost differences for different levels of episode severity, much like the health status adjustment addressed in the capitation section. Furthermore, not all the care patients receive neatly fits into a "bundle." In addition, managing episode-based compensation can be more complex than working it under the simpler FFS and capitation models.

The Health Insurance Portability and Accountability Act's (HIPAA) provisions, along with Medicare and Medicaid, are now in effect

What is the purpose of HIPAA?

HIPAA, officially known as Public Law 104-191, serves two main objectives: it continues to cover employees with health insurance whether they move jobs or lose their jobs, and it eventually lowers healthcare costs by standardizing the electronic transmission of administrative and financial activities. Increasing access to long-term care services and insurance is another goal, along with reducing instances of abuse, fraud, and waste in the delivery of healthcare and insurance.

Government-run health plans and healthcare organizations are required by the HIPAA Privacy Rule to adhere to similar privacy protection standards to those that apply to private organizations. For instance, government-run health plans like Medicare and Medicaid are required to take the same safeguards as private insurance plans or health maintenance organizations in order to protect the claims and health information they receive from beneficiaries (HMOs). Additionally, the Privacy Act of 1974, which limits the disclosure of personal information about citizens to other government agencies and the general public, must also be complied with by all federal agencies.

The sole additional power granted to the government relates to the Privacy Rule's provisions for protection. The Rule requires that health plans, hospitals, and other covered entities cooperate with the efforts of the Office for Civil Rights (OCR) of the Department of Health and Human Services (HHS) to investigate complaints or otherwise ensure compliance. This is done to ensure that covered entities protect the privacy of patients as is required.

Explain the process for preparing invoices for procedures rendered

It might be challenging to translate patient notes into claims. It's not simple to process claims, either. Before you reach the collection stage, it may take weeks and several communications. It would help if you created consistent workflows because of this. To expedite billing tasks, adhere to the crucial steps in the medical billing procedure listed below.

Step 1: Register Patients

The first stage is obtaining the patient personal and insurance data, such as name, age, residence, contact information, policy number, and insurance provider. Create checklists to ensure that you don't leave out any vital inputs in the process of collecting them. You need to look over the intake forms before you file anything. Check for any data that is either missing or unreadable before validating the insurance information. These days, the majority of clinics use electronic medical records, electronic health records, or medical billing technology to streamline the data-collecting activities.

Registration for new patients can be a hassle. Clients are required to wait before they even start receiving care. You can increase patient satisfaction by putting pre-registration strategies into practice. Patients favored an online or mobile-enabled registration experience, 64 percent of clinicians noticed in a survey by Experian Health. The process of registering new patients can be simplified with the appointment of a new patient coordinator, abbreviated as NPC.

Step 2: Verify Insurance Plans

Each company has a different insurance coverage policy. For instance, most health plan sponsors do not pay for aesthetic operations. Consequently, establishing financial responsibility is essential.

The following methods exist for determining insurance eligibility.

You can reach insurance professionals by calling Payers. To find the providers' phone numbers, get information from patient files. Make sure that you are chatting with the right representative by checking. To guarantee HIPAA-compliant communication, the rep may occasionally ask you to provide information about your practice. The operator will disclose patients' insurance information after establishing a secure connection.

Health plan firms now use interactive voice response (IVR) systems to free up sales representatives' time for other crucial activities. Using the touch-tone keypad, the interactive voice response system (IVR) will present you with a menu of possibilities from which you can select one. The system will direct your call to a particular professional or department if you require additional information.

Online Lookup

Don't want to spend all day on the phone? Through the websites of payers, you can get online materials for eligibility. You might need to fill out various forms or browse directories to find the relevant data.

Leverage Digital Solutions

You can run real-time eligibility checks with some billing tools to let clients know about out-of-pocket costs. The advantages of using software to check insurance coverage are noted below:

- Verify several insurances at once.
- Boost interaction with patients.
- Decrease denials.
- Up the amount collected.
- Spend less on administration.

You can include the following items in your verification checklist:

- The policy's start and end dates.
- Details regarding patient deductibles.
- Coverage restrictions.
- Copay specifics.
- Requirements for documentation.

Patients also have a lot going on in their lives. They might forget to keep you updated on any changes that have been made to the health plan. You must constantly recheck insurance policies as a result.

Step 3: Create Superbills

A superbill is essentially a thorough invoice that condenses the services that were actually rendered into one document. They can send this invoice to their insurance company so that it can be paid for.

Verify the latest client file information if they frequently visit your office. Additionally, request official identification like a passport or driver's license. Copayments can be obtained either before or after the visit. It relies on the policy of your practice. You must write the medical report and transmit it to the medical coder once the client leaves the store. After that, the coder will transform the data into diagnosis and procedure codes. You can now construct a superbill for the client that includes their demographic information, medical information, and insurance information.

Step 4: Generate and Transmit Claims

After you have successfully created a superbill, the next step is to either manually or electronically submit a medical claim. To prevent denials, don't forget to review your document for coding and formatting issues. Each claim must include information about the patient and the procedures (CPT or HCPCS codes). After then, the requirement from a clinical standpoint can be demonstrated by combining these procedural codes with a diagnosis code (an ICD code).

Claims must also include information about insurance providers identified by their National Provider Identifiers (NPI) numbers. It is imperative that the regulations laid down by the Office of the Inspector General (OIG) and the Health Insurance Portability and Accountability Act (HIPAA) be adhered to. Either through clearinghouses or directly to payers, claims can be submitted. Claims are reformatted and checked for mistakes by a clearinghouse. Then they deliver them to health insurance providers.

Step 5: Monitor Adjudication

Payers analyze claims during adjudication to determine whether they are valid or not. Claims are either approved, denied, or rejected by insurance companies.

Case 1: Acceptance of the Claim by Payers

Insurance firms approve legitimate claims that don't contain any code, documentation, or data input problems. After the claim has been validated, you will receive a statement known as an explanation of benefits (EOB). The patient's name, the payee's name, the policy number, and the services covered are all listed on this paper. Remember that the insurance company will only make payments following the terms of the contract with the patient.

Case 2: If Payers Disapprove of the Claim

A claim will be rejected and returned to you if it is incomplete or incorrectly coded. In certain circumstances, you can amend your claim and submit it again. A decision that was made by the insurance company might be challenged by you in the form of an appeal. You are within your rights to request an evaluation from a third party as well. The health insurance provider will cover the cost of the treatments or services provided if a third-party reviewer determines in the client's favor.

Case 3: If Payers Reject the Claim

Insurance companies reject claims when the client's health plan doesn't cover a specific procedure. In such cases, you might resend the claim to the payer after checking it for errors. You must tell the patient about their financial responsibilities if the claim is again refused.

These processes can take longer than usual. You should contact insurance providers again to inquire about the adjudication status.

Step 6: Prepare patient statements.

The document in question is a bill that details all of the procedures or services that the client received. Additionally, you can include an explanation of the benefits statement with the invoice to give patients an explanation of why certain services are covered and others are not. Take a look at the table that follows to get a better understanding of the differences between a billing statement and an explanation of benefits.

Step 7: Handle Collections

Sending patient statements through mail completes the process. If your customers do not pay their invoices by the due date, you are required to initiate the follow-up steps. When handling collections gets difficult, you can enlist collection agencies. Before retaliating against clients, don't forget to review your company's collection policies.

Front-End **Medical Billing**

Medical billing begins when patients check in at the hospital or office and make appointments. Staff from the administration make sure that patients fill out the required paperwork and provide patient information during pre-registration. This information consists of things like a home address and insurance coverage. After confirming the patient's health plan coverage, the staff verifies the patient's financial responsibilities.

The staff informs the patients of potential fees incurred during the front-end billing procedure. Typically, while scheduling appointments, offices can accept copayments from clients. Coders receive the medical records from the check-out patients and translate the data into codes.

Back-End Billing

The fundamentals of medical billing also cover back-end billing. Medical billers and coders create the "superbill" using patient data and codes. Knowing what a "superbill" is in this context is crucial. A provider uses it as a particular form for submitting claims. Usually, this form contains:

- Provider details
- data regarding patients
- data regarding patients

A clinician may also include remarks or notes to support the need for medically necessary care. Billers use information from the superbill to prepare claims. Billers frequently work with the CMS-1500, CMS-1450, or UB-04 forms.

Every trustworthy medical billing company can submit claims without making any mistakes. The most critical medical billing fundamentals that medical billers must comprehend are front-end and back-end billing. Without thoroughly learning these procedures, it is hard to guarantee dependable medical billing services.

Payment Posting

What does medical billing payment posting entail?

Payment posting is the act of viewing payments and a medical practice's overall financial picture. Additionally, it alludes to recording payments in the medical billing program. It offers a perspective on patient payments, insurance checks from ERAs, and insurance payments in EOBs. Understanding the financial picture can help you identify income leakage and take fast action to fix them.

What makes the medical billing procedure crucial?

Any medical practice cannot function without a proper medical billing system. Your revenue depends on how precise and effective your billing procedure is. A medical approach is able to collect appropriate compensation for the services it provides as a result of the process. That is how doctors, nurses, and other healthcare professionals are compensated.

How crucial is precise payment posting?

Since there are several processes involved in the medical billing process and numerous claims are handled daily, problems are expected. Because of this, difficulties can be significantly decreased by paying attention to the entire procedure. Your payment posters will be attentive in identifying patterns behind denials for medical necessity, uncovered treatments, and prior authorizations if your team executes its job correctly. Additionally, they must escalate any problems to other coding and billing team members so they can be resolved. Additionally, the entire process runs more smoothly for everyone involved, including the front and back office workers.

How does the revenue cycle relate to payment posting?

Whether you utilize an internal billing system or a third-party billing service, payment posting should be a crucial aspect of the revenue cycle.

By keeping an eye out for familiar patterns within your business. Putting a proper method in place is crucial because payment posting has excellent potential to increase revenues and improve the entire medical billing process.

How to evaluate the payment posting process

- Receiving payments in the form of checks doesn't guarantee that everything is going smoothly. Even so, you should continue to assess your payment posting procedure routinely. Here are some pointers for thorough reviewing.
- beginning with your crew
- Your workers should be the starting point for any review of your payment posting procedure. You need the appropriate staff in sufficient numbers. Staffing levels should be determined by volume rather than just the number of practitioners who just happen to be employed at the practice.
- It pays to have the correct employees and a sufficient number of them. Given the volume of payments most practices receive, accuracy and productivity are crucial during the billing process. Therefore, when recruiting posters, take the time to check references, and trust your gut when interviewing individuals.

What are the proper procedures for posting payments in medical billing?

The revenue cycle's payment posting phase is crucial. You have the choice of utilizing an internal billing solution or contracting it out to a third party. Here are some steps you may do to make sure a precise payment posting is made:

Always check to see if the data on EOBs and ERAs corresponds to the payments.

Examine potential problems or revenue cycle leakage when collecting deductibles or copayments while processing insurance remittances.

To prevent mistakes, let management know if any critical medical services, non-covered services, or prior permission requests are denied.

Always follow up on rejections effectively.

The implication of overall efficiency and infrastructure is accurate payment posting.

How health insurance claims get paid

Health insurance has two different types: defined benefit plans and indemnity plans. An indemnity plan allows you to make a claim for reimbursement of actual out-of-pocket expenses, up to the maximum amount of coverage provided by the plan, provided that the policy's terms and conditions are met. A defined benefit insurance plan protects you financially in the event that you are diagnosed with one of the predetermined illnesses.

You will receive the sum insured if you have a contract for any of them and can show valid proof. In this case, subject to the terms and circumstances of the insurance, payment of the sum insured is not tied to any expenses incurred but rather to getting the sickness.

The indemnity cover, also referred to as medical, is typically purchased. This article discusses how an indemnity policy pays out on insurance. An indemnity-type health insurance claim is often paid in two ways: repayment of expenses or cashless hospital services.

Hospital cashless services

A list of hospitals included in the network will be sent to you by your insurer when you purchase a health insurance plan. You can utilize cashless perks if you receive treatment at these institutions. In these affiliated hospitals, you can present your insurance e-card and continue your hospitalization without spending any cash. The only other requirement is that your health insurance policy must cover the ailment or illness, subject to the amount of coverage you have. When a patient is discharged, the hospital will submit all of the necessary invoices to the insurance company. And following completion of the cost analysis, the insurer will pay the bill.

Reimbursement of expenses

The reimbursement method is the alternative to using your health insurance. You can pay your medical bills up front, receive treatment, and then submit all your receipts to your insurance company. The insurance reimburses you for the costs incurred after evaluating the statements by your sum assured limit. The payment mechanism kicks in if an insured individual has to be admitted to a hospital that is not part of their network or affiliation due to an unexpected medical emergency.

When can you file a claim?

To be eligible for benefits under most health insurance plans, a patient must be admitted for at least 24 hours or longer. This is true except for a few specific daycare operations listed in your policy guidelines. It's also crucial to confirm the legitimacy of your health insurance policy. Make sure your coverage has not expired so you can submit claims.

Even if reading through an insurance policy's terminology can be tedious, you still need to be aware of some critical points. Important insurance information includes specific operations limitations, room rent ceilings, waiting periods for particular ailments, co-pays, and exclusions from coverage. Typically, waiting periods apply to specific illnesses or disorders under health insurance programs. A claim for a disease or medical condition still inside the waiting period may not be honored by your insurer. They will periodically send you insurance cards if you rely on your company to offer your health insurance. It is imperative to carry the most recent version of the card because an older card might no longer be valid.

How to get your claims paid

You will likely visit an insurance desk at almost all network facilities throughout your hospital stay. For planned hospitalization, you must fill out a pre-approval form at the counter to use the cashless service. Within 24 hours of admission, notification for an emergency hospitalization can be made. For a cashless claim to be accepted, only the insured's identity evidence and health card are required. Simply fill out the pre-approval paperwork provided by the hospital's insurance desk, and the third-party administrator (TPA) desk will take care of the remainder of the documents.

You should discuss the specifics of your policy coverage with the hospital as soon as possible. This will prevent misunderstandings, and the hospital personnel will contact you if the insurance coverage expires. You must consider variables unique to reimbursement to ensure the seamless operation of your reimbursement claim. For a hassle-free experience, you must give a wide variety of papers. Documents such as a properly completed claim form signed by the policyholder, a doctor's recommendation for admission, the complete breakdown of the hospital's final bill, and the original invoices and receipts for pre- and post-hospitalization costs.

All original hospital bills that have been signed and adequately stamped must be collected. Along with any further research and test information, you must also submit all doctor records, including diagnoses, admissions, and report details. The discharge summary is a critical document for a reimbursement request. Do not overlook the importance of including it with your claim. Although you must submit the originals, having a copy of each document on hand can be helpful.

After reviewing and accepting the claim, your insurer will transfer the money to the account information specified in the forms. Therefore, before submitting the paperwork, make sure you have entered the correct information and double-check it. In addition to the know-your-customer (KYC) documents the policyholder has to supply, you are also required to provide a canceled check. In this manner, claims will be settled more quickly, and there will be fewer chances of a claim being denied.

Medical Billing and Coding Salaries

Although medical billing and coding specialists have separate skill sets and duties, they are categorized as medical records and health information technicians and make about the same amount of money. Ninety-seven percent of respondents said they made between $29,430 and $274,50. A report published last year states that the top 10 AAPC programmers' salaries differ by 33%. The average pay of 66.752 would increase with a second certification.

Build skills with stackable degrees

It is unnecessary to wait four years before adding this qualification to your resume. Many line programs are designed for stacking. You can start with fewer credentials if you enroll in a stackable program, such as the Undergraduate Certificate in Medical Billing and Coding. You have access to a wide variety of online training courses that can assist you in strengthening your professional abilities.

What you'll learn in a medical Coding and Billing Program

Because they have comparable jobs, several schools combine medical billing and coding into a single course with dual certifications. Both medical billing and medical coding certificates require students to understand federal coding standards. Students who select only one method of study might choose from various programs.

How can I learn more about medical coding and billing in the quickest and most efficient way possible?

It would seem that there are many more reasons to finish your medical billing and coding career. The results of a relatively modest amount of effort can yield considerable benefits as well as career stability. Professional organizations that encourage professional development are the best places to go for detailed information on these concerns.

Chapter 5: The Importance of People Skills for Coding and Billing Specialists in the Medical Industry

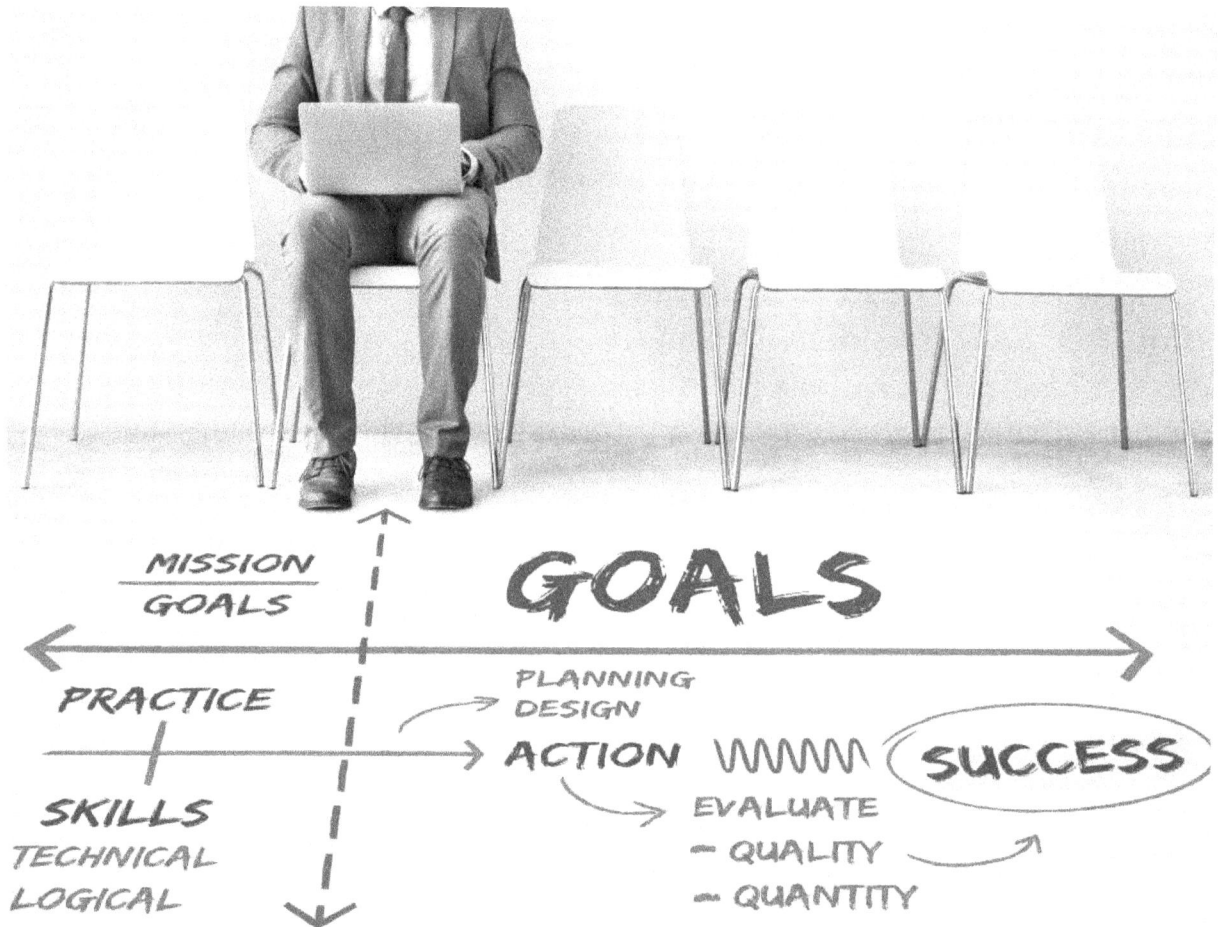

When you think about core competencies for the industry, such as knowing how to use coding software, being familiar with the International Classification of Diseases (ICD) database, and Current Procedural Terminology (CPT), and having a fundamental understanding of finance and healthcare, medical billing and coding are probably the first things that come to mind.

However, those are not the only skills that come in handy when it comes to medical coding and billing. Both seasoned professionals and those who are just beginning their careers in a given industry might benefit from developing their soft skills.

Soft skills might even improve your ability to carry out the many duties of your profession, such as your capacity to handle payment negotiations and claim processes correctly.

Here are five soft skills that medical billers and coders absolutely must possess.

1. Communication Skills

Specialists in medical billing often contact various individuals, including doctors, nurses, patients, and insurance companies.

For the purposes of precisely completing a patient's record for the purpose of coding, obtaining pre-authorization for referrals, or following up with insurance companies and patients on outstanding bills, clear communication is essential. For instance, the medical biller must comprehend the problem, investigate the claim, and effectively present the evidence if the insurance company denies the claim.

You will need to respond to inquiries, clarify fees, interpret policies, and assist customers in taking the following steps to advance the billing process, regardless of who you communicate with.

2. Active Listening

Being sensitive to the other person's requirements is essential for effective communication. Active listening is critical for complex billing, coding, and payment procedures that frequently involve several parties.

When working with healthcare experts, please pay close attention to how they carry out the operations you are coding so that you can accurately apply the proper codes. Active listening can also be beneficial when you need to contact an insurance provider to find out why a claim was rejected and find a solution.

Last but not least, the capacity to hear patients out and comprehend their circumstances (such as when they're having difficulties paying their bills) will aid you in finding solutions that benefit both the patient and the healthcare practitioner.

3. Problem-Solving Skills

Specialists in medical billing and coding do more than just match codes to procedures and generate invoices. They also cooperate with insurance providers to resolve disputes or provide solutions for claims that have been rejected. During the billing process, medical billers and coders must be able to speak with patients in a straightforward and considerate manner.

As a medical biller and coder, you should approach each problem to resolve it or do everything you can to improve the patient's situation. If a claim is denied, for example, you need to be able to use the tools available to you to hunt for evidence that will convince the insurance company to accept the claim anyhow.

Although the dynamics are different when working with patients, you still need to be skilled at problem-solving. Some patients might not have enough money to pay a bill in full. When that occurs, you will need to collaborate with them to create a payment strategy that benefits your care facility and its financial situation.

4. Conflict Management

Negotiating payments with patients can lead to unpleasant and emotionally charged situations. In order to devise a solution that is beneficial to the patient and does not put the practice's financial viability in jeopardy, medical billers need to be able to think rapidly while maintaining their composure.

Medical billers and coders need to be quick on their feet, inventive, and knowledgeable about policy and procedure to help in these circumstances. For instance, you should know the various payment plan structures, how to negotiate with insurance providers, and how to submit claims for the best results.

This talent can be developed in two ways: through experience and through being able to adapt to the needs of the patient. Pay close attention, and show empathy. Don't assume anything; instead, take the time to learn about each person's particular circumstance.

5. Attention to Detail

Medical coders must precisely identify each process step and connect it with a billing code. Medical billers, meantime, must make sure that each payment and invoice corresponds to the relevant information.

Attention helps avoid sending incorrect codes to insurance companies and sluggish claim processing. It can help reduce payment inconsistencies caused by incorrectly entering numbers into coding and billing software.

Medical billers and coders must be meticulous in spotting coding errors to collect the correct income and clear up problems with bookkeeping and tax data problems.

6. Organization Skills

Medical coders and billers frequently deal with the data for numerous cases and patients at once. In order to do a good job at your job, you need to have the ability to retrieve information both accurately and swiftly.

When a patient or insurance company calls, you should be able to access claim information rapidly. You should also be able to maintain track of payments and unpaid balances to support your billing department. When things get busy, you can save time and be more productive by creating an organized system for yourself that makes it possible to access information rapidly. Additionally, you must maintain a list of patient information and ensure its security due to increasingly strict data protection requirements.

If you are in charge of preparing financial statements, it is quite essential that you keep all of the financial information organized. Instead of rushing to gather data every time you need it, a well-organized system enables you to ensure your reports' accuracy better.

7. Time Management

The majority of medical billers and coders are independent contractors, which provides them with a great deal of leeway on how and when they carry out their jobs.

Your workload and work schedule must be disciplined because your workday will be less structured. Professionals who work in medical billing and coding are responsible for a wide array of tasks. The burden can quickly increase if you don't understand the steps necessary and how long it will take you to complete each task.

Some employees may lose up to 40% of their working time when switching jobs. To remain productive, assess your workload. Then, you can combine related tasks to attract more attention and hasten the process.

8. Multitasking

It can be challenging yet frequently required to switch between jobs fast. Medical billers and coders must be able to change their attention often throughout the day to deal with incoming requests, tasks, or inquiries.

Take the situation where you are in the middle of sending out invoices, and the phone rings. Additionally, you must be able to respond swiftly and accurately if an insurance company requests information before going back to your original activity.

Fortunately, you can learn how to multitask. Try organizing and prioritizing related items on your to-do list to test if you can complete chores more quickly. Then, log your time.

9. Adaptivity and Agility

Today's medical billers and coders must be able to deal with healthcare technology that is rapidly expanding, as well as have a firm understanding of new diagnoses and available treatments. You'll also need to understand ever-evolving insurance laws, government-funded initiatives, and data privacy laws.

For instance, the implementation of ICD-11 necessitates learning a new coding system and using new diagnostic codes by medical coding professionals. You might need to adapt to new workflows because ICD-11 allows for more connectivity with other technologies, such as EHR systems.

Every workplace provides a variety of services and operates uniquely. Medical coding and billing professionals must be quick learners and ready to adapt to new procedures.

10. Collaboration and Teamwork

You must communicate effectively with various people to do your job well, whether you operate as the sole medical billing and coding professional in a small care facility or as a freelance consultant.

In a more extensive facility, you'll probably collaborate with several other personnel, such as other medical coders and billers. You might need to contact a few medical specialists engaged in the treatment process to double-check information when following up with patients or looking into claims. Working well with others and communicating effectively can go a long way toward fostering a cooperative atmosphere and assisting you in your work duties more effectively.

11. Empathy and Compassion

The technical and mathematical aspects of medical billing and coding are straightforward to become engrossed in. Having said that, the ability to interact with patients is as as important as having technical understanding.

Patients' life and finances may be strained by the high cost of treating a chronic illness. To successfully negotiate payment with patients, you must understand their points of view and make them feel as though you are on their side.

Empathy is essential for workers in the healthcare industry, as they are the ones providing direct care to patients. Medical billing and coding specialists should use their knowledge and abilities to represent patients better, understand insurance rules and increase the number of paid claims.

12. Proactivity and Self-Motivation

As was mentioned earlier, the majority of medical billers and coders are able to function on their own. It is frequently your obligation to ensure that tasks are finished in a timely manner while causing as little disruption as possible.

Be proactive in positioning yourself for success to manage your duties and perform at a high level. You can set up a system to assist you in keeping track of payments, following up on claims, and resolving inconsistencies. You can think about contacting the other parties directly to ensure the prompt resolution of any concerns rather than waiting for patients or insurance companies to call.

For internal communications, the same holds. You can prevent delays later in the billing process by speaking with medical experts on concerns or omissions on a claim.

13. A Positive Attitude

Everyone can benefit from a positive outlook, but medical billing and coding professionals who frequently interact with many people may find it helpful.

Being positive can help you communicate with coworkers more efficiently or face problematic contact with patients or staff from insurance companies. Positivity can help you manage stress and support you in getting through challenging and complex situations.

Chapter 6: You Should Be Familiar with These Common Medical Billing and Insurance Terms

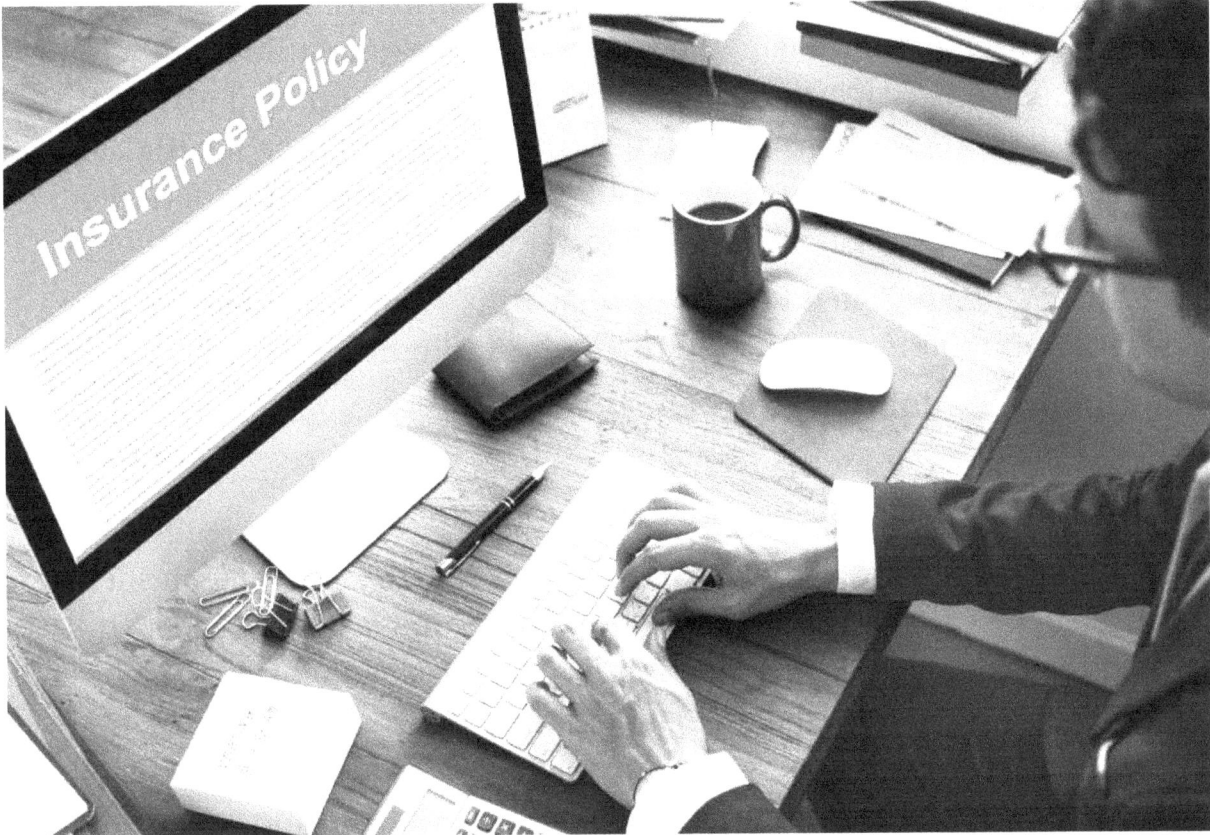

Do you find yourself juggling a significant amount of paper work? Are you having trouble with the billing for your eye care and medical optometry services? Do you need a refresher course on standard insurance and medical billing phrases? To assist you in increasing collections, avoiding having claims rejected or refused, and concentrating on increasing revenue for your eye care business, we have you covered with a dictionary of insurance terminology and billing advice.

What is an Adjudication Date in Medical Billing

Every hospital in the medical field depends on insurance companies to pay for the medical care provided to their covered patients. Therefore, the hospital must submit medical claims to the insurance company each time an insured patient visits the hospital for treatment. Medical claims are now submitted electronically to simplify, speed up, and efficiently complete the process. After receiving the claims from the healthcare provider, the insurance company will spend some time conducting an investigation into them. The adjudication date plays a role in this.

It's crucial to comprehend the meaning of the term "adjudication date" before moving on to the concept of "claims adjudication."

The Claims Evaluation Procedure

Five steps are taken by the insurance company when deciding on claims:

1. Initial Processing Review: This process examines information such as the patient's name (in case it is misspelled), the patient's gender (if it differs from the identification number), the plan number or member ID, the date of service, and the service codes.
2. Information that is checked automatically includes things like invalid diagnostic and procedure codes, invalid pre-authorizations, invalid certifications, claims that are submitted after the deadline, and patient eligibility (for claim mismatches, inactive/terminated coverage, missed payments, and so on).
3. Manual Review: Skilled examiners of medical and health care claims perform manual reviews of claims. When deciding if surgery is necessary, a patient's medical records may be requested and examined for any unlisted procedures. Any inconsistency in the information could render the claim invalid.
4. Payment Determination: Whether or not the reimbursement should be granted depends on the outcome of this phase. If such is the case, how much of the money needs to be repaid? The payment could either be made, be denied, or be reduced. These are the three possible possibilities.
5. Money: Finally, the medical office is paid by the insurance company

for the services they provided. The word "explanation of payment" or "remittance guidance" are both terminology that are used to describe this payment. Remittance advice outlines the justifications for any adjustments and reductions in cost, denials, or uncovered expenses. It contains information regarding, among other things, the allowed amount, the approved amount, the covered amount, the adjudication date, the paid amount, and the patient responsibility amount.

For the medical office to receive full payment, it must ensure that all the information is entered accurately (or allowed). A single mistake in the submitted claim could invalidate it and cause it to be denied. Utilizing a clearinghouse or medical billing company's outsourcing of medical billing services is the best approach to filing a medical claim free of errors. This enables the hospital to obtain the support of skilled medical billers to file claims that are as accurate as possible.

Chapter 7: Medical Billing Terms and Descriptions for Billers and Coders

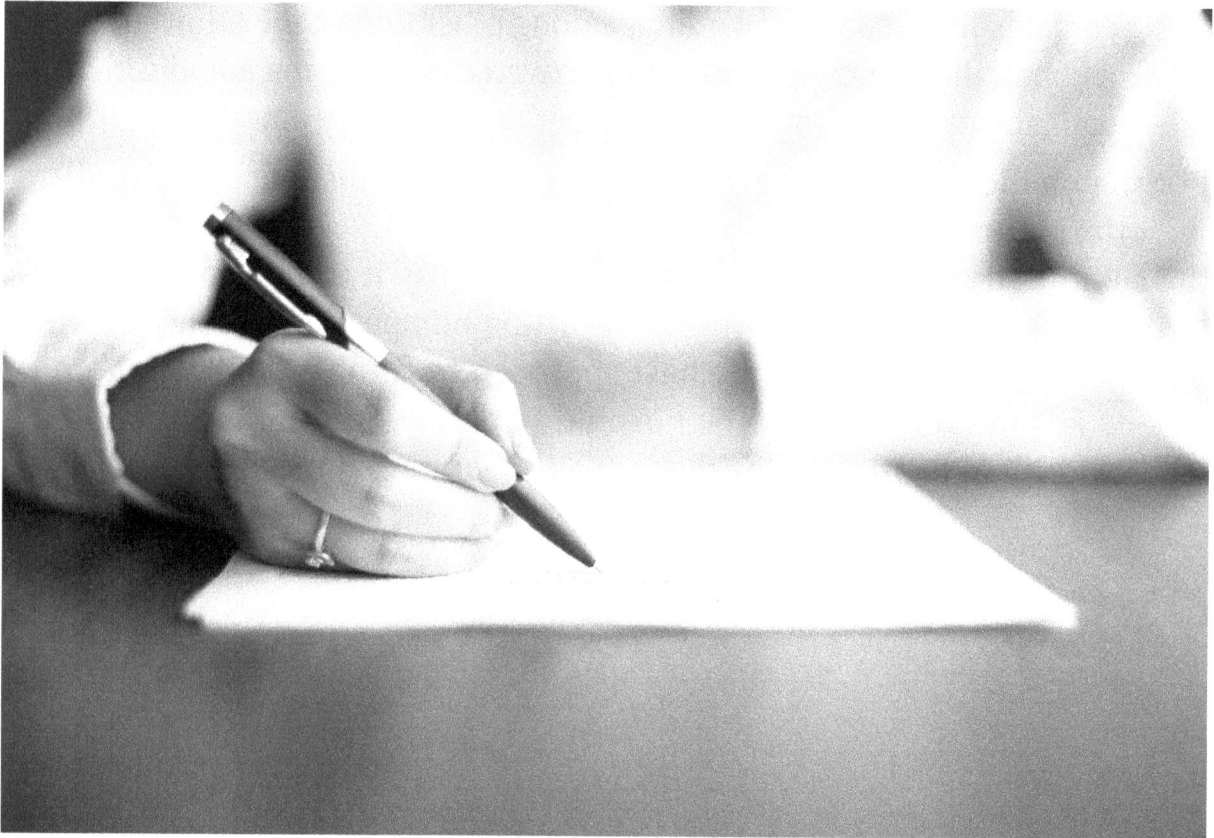

Accounts Receivable (AR): Whether the patient is financially responsible or their insurance provider is, a medical account receivable is the unpaid compensation owing to providers for rendered treatments and services.

Adjudication: Examining medical claims for the appropriate information before issuing the payment is referred to as claims adjudication. The purpose is to evaluate the integrity of the filed lawsuit, judge it, and then approve or reject the reimbursement in light of the outcome.

Advance Beneficiary Notice of Noncoverage (ABN): A permission form alerts the patient that if their insurance company rejects the claim, they might be financially responsible for the costs. Before you give the patient any non-covered services or goods, the patient must fill out and sign the ABN.

Aging Bucket or AR Aging: Accounts receivable aging, often known as "aging bucket" or "AR aging," is a periodic report that classifies a company's accounts receivable based on how long an invoice has been past due. It serves as a barometer to assess the stability and dependability of a company's clientele.

A warning indicator that business may be slowing down or that the company is taking on more credit risk in its sales practices is when a company's receivables are being collected significantly more slowly than usual.

Allowed Amount: The most money an insurance company will permit a provider to charge for a healthcare service that qualifies. This sum may be covered by the insurance, the patient, or a combination of both, depending on the patient's specific coverage.

Applied to Deductible (ATD): The sum of expenses a patient must cover before their insurance company begins to pay (Applied to Deductible, or ATD). The patient insurance statement typically contains this information.

Assignment of Benefits (AOB): When a patient signs documents directing his health insurance company to pay his doctor or hospital directly, this is known as an assignment of benefits.

Authorization: Asking your health insurance provider or plan to consider a decision or a complaint. An insurance or health plan's approval of services, such as hospitalization, is known as authorization. Before receiving treatment, your health plan or insurer may demand pre-authorization. The sum is shown on the billing statement as owed to Mayo Clinic.

Authorization Number: The therapy or service has been authorized by the patient's insurance plan, according to the authorization number.

A payment arrangement known as "bundling" is one in which you receive care from numerous healthcare specialists treating you for the same or related problems. Instead of paying each of these professionals separately for each treatment, test, or procedure, you pay for the bundle as a whole.

Claim Adjustment Reason Codes (CARCs): In order to effectively communicate an adjustment, claim adjustment reason codes, also known as CARCs, must provide an explanation for why a claim or service line was paid differently than it was invoiced for. An adjustment reason code won't be if a claim or bar isn't adjusted.

Clearinghouse: A middleman or intermediary regularly communicates eye care providers' financial information and secure, HIPAA-compliant electronic medical claims to one or more payers in batch transactions. Medicare, Medicaid, Managed Care, private insurance, and other third-party payers are payers.

Charge Entry: Before you submit a vision plan or health insurance claim, you must first enter accurate medical billing information and assign diagnostic codes, procedure codes, and modifiers. A single error could result in a claim being rejected or refused, costing thousands of dollars in revenue.

Claim Adjustment Group Codes: On the Explanation of Benefits (EOB) or the Electronic Remittance Advice, you'll see these codes, which consist of two alphabetic characters and represent the point of contact for a claim adjustment, respectively (ERA). These group codes include a claim adjustment reason code, either a numeric or alpha-numeric code, that explains why a claim or service line was paid (or not paid) differently from how it had been billed.

Claim Scrubbing: The process of checking your practice's medical claims for problems that can lead payers (i.e., insurance companies) to reject the claim is known as claim scrubbing. Claim scrubbers check the Current Procedural Terminology (CPT) codes on your claims, whether they are people or computer programs (we'll discuss both in a moment).

CMS-1500 02/12 Form: Use the CMS-1500 02/12 Form, which may be found on the website of the Centers for Medicare and Medicaid Services, to submit paper claims to Medicare and Medicaid (CMS). It's possible that the red ink will identify the form. An HCFA form is another term for the Health Care Financing Administration (HCFA), which was the prior name for the Centers for Medicare and Medicaid Services.

Coordination of Benefits: The phrase "coordination of benefits" (COB) refers to the process by which Medicare-eligible individuals' health and prescription insurance plans decide who is responsible for paying what amounts.

Co-insurance: The portion of a covered health care service's cost you are responsible for paying (20%, for example) after your deductible has been met. The most a plan will spend on a covered medical service. Alternatively known as "negotiated rate," "payment allowance," or "qualifying expense."

Co-payment (Co-pay): You pay a set fee ($20, for instance) for a covered medical procedure once your deductible has been met. The most a plan will spend on a covered medical service. Alternatively known as "negotiated rate," "payment allowance," or "qualifying expense."

Credentialing: Also known as credentialing of healthcare providers. This is how the qualifications of a doctor are gathered and authenticated (verified) (professional background and educational history). Credentialing ensures that healthcare professionals have the necessary credentials, licenses, and training to offer patient care. "Getting on insurance panels" is another term for the process of insurance plan credentialing.

Current Procedural Terminology (CPT®) Code: The American Medical Association® developed a system of codes that consist of several categories and types of five-digit codes as well as two-character modifiers that can be used to identify any adjustments that were made to the surgery. A fifth alpha character, such as F, T, or U, may be present in some codes. Category I, Category II, Category II, and Proprietary Laboratory Analyses (PLA) codes are the four categories of CPT codes.

Date of Service (DOS): The date of the treatment, also known as the "Date of Service" (DOS). Diagnosis Code (ICD-10): The ICD-10-CM diagnostic code, also known as the International Classification of Diseases, is used to characterize patients' conditions as well as their diagnoses. This is in contrast to the ICD-10-PCS code, which is used to define inpatient operations. The diagnosis code gives the person paying for the service an explanation of why the service was performed.

Denied Claim: The insurance company or third-party payer has already received and processed the claim; it has undergone the adjudication procedure. However, even if a payer rejects a claim, you can still appeal the denial because it doesn't always mean the claim isn't valid.

Effective Date: The day an insurance benefits contract takes effect.

EDI Enrollment: Enroll in an EDI clearinghouse or with specific payers so you can submit claims electronically. You must enroll with your clearinghouse when you set up your billing system. You can send and receive remits connected to your Tax ID using each clearinghouse's specific submitter and receiver IDs. Before you can submit claims to some payers via the clearinghouse, such as Medicare and Medicaid, you must complete enrollment papers.

Electronic Data Interchange (EDI): Your billing system and the insurance provider's relationship is mediated through electronic data interchange (EDI), which is how billing distributes claim data to different insurance payers.

Electronic Funds Transfer (EFT): Insurance settlement payments can now be electronically deposited (EFT), which is akin to direct deposit, to your bank account. Many insurance payers increasingly insist that providers accept EFT payments in order to keep up with the demands of the provider network.

Medicare Advantage Plans: Private companies that have received Medicare's permission offer Medicare Advantage, a specific sort of Medicare health plan. They are an alternative to the traditional Medicare program and provide coverage for all of the costs that are associated with Medicare. They provide the same hospital coverage under Part A and medical coverage under Part B, but they do not cover hospice care.

Medicare Beneficiary Identifier (MBI): On the patient's Medicare card, the Social Security Number (SSN)-based Health Insurance Claim Number is replaced with the Medicare Beneficiary Identity (MBI), which is an 11-character alphanumeric identifier (HICN).

Medicare Administrative Contractor (MAC): Beneficiaries of Medicare

are represented by a private healthcare insurance during the claims processing procedure.

Medicare Beneficiary Identifier (MBI): On the patient's Medicare card, the patient's Health Insurance Claim Number, which is based on their Social Security Number (SSN), will be replaced with the Medicare Beneficiary Identifier (MBI), which is an 11-character alphanumeric number (HICN).

Medically Necessary: According to Medicare, medically necessary treatments or supplies are those that "meet accepted standards of medicine" and are required to diagnose or treat sickness, injury, condition, disease, or one of its symptoms.

National Provider Identifier (NPI): a one-of-a-kind identifying number consisting of 10 digits that is assigned to healthcare practitioners and is needed under HIPAA. The National Plan and Provider Enumeration System is the entity that provided the provider with this number (NPPES).

Electronic Remittance Advice (ERA): The term "electronic remittance advice" refers to either an electronic data interchange (EDI) or a transaction that takes place entirely online and transmits claim details (ERA). ERAs are typically used in order to do tasks such as automatically posting claim payments into the billing system.

Eligibility and Verification: Verification of eligibility ensures the insurance information is accurate and aids in calculating how much a patient might owe (e.g., co-pays, co-insurance, and deductibles). Giving your clients more precise cost estimates will increase patient satisfaction and prevent more claim denials.

Evaluation and Management (E/M) Codes: When a doctor or other healthcare professional invoices for their services, they use a series of CPT® codes called the Evaluation and Management (E/M) codes to designate various patient visits. These medical codes are applicable to new patients as well as existing patients for office visits and services that involve "evaluating and managing" patient health. E/M coding is broken down into three distinct parts: the history, the medical decision-making (MDM), and the examination.

Benefits Explanation (EOB): After processing the claim, the insurance company sends a letter called an explanation of benefits (EOB) to the provider. The EOB also shows the proper amount, non-covered charges, the amount paid to the provider, any co-pays, co-insurance, and deductibles that are the patient's responsibility, in addition to the total costs (amount billed).

Fee Schedule: The fee schedule that is part of the contract between the insurance company and the provider details the services for which the insurance company is willing to pay (the permitted amount) (except Medicare and Medicaid).

Global Period: A time frame following a surgical treatment in which the original surgery code includes some follow-up procedures. The worldwide period could be 0 days, ten days, or 90 days, depending on the surgery. When operations that would typically be included in the routine follow-up care are carried out for unrelated reasons within this time, specific modifiers may be used.

Guarantor: The person who is in charge of making the payment and is responsible for it. They are sometimes referred to as the accountable party as well.

Healthcare Common Procedure Coding System (HCPCS): The Healthcare Common Procedure Coding System, also known as HCPCS, is a standardized code system that is required for medical providers to use in order to submit healthcare claims to Medicare and other health insurances in a manner that is consistent and orderly. The HCPCS consists of two different sets of medical codes: HCPCS Level I and HCPCS Level II.

Modifier: Modifiers are added to the Healthcare Common Procedure Coding System (HCPCS) or Current Procedural Terminology (CPT®) codes to provide additional information required for processing a claim, such as describing the rationale behind a physician or other qualified healthcare professional performing a particular service and procedure.

National Correct Coding Initiative (NCCI) Edits: NCCI edits stop bundling and unbundling caused by improper use of HCPCS billing codes and CPT® procedure codes, including combining inappropriate code combinations.

National Coverage Determination (NCD): A usage management technique known as National Coverage Determination (NCD) determines whether Medicare will cover a particular commodity or service.

HIPAA: The federal statute known as the Health Insurance Portability and Accountability Act (HIPAA) has been in effect since 1996. Three key responsibilities—confidentiality, integrity, and availability—emphasize HIPAA compliance. HIPAA safeguards the confidentiality of personally identifiable protected health information (PHI), offers physical and technological protection for PHI, and streamlines billing and other electronic transactions.

ICD-10 Codes: Tenth Revision of the International Classification of Diseases. While ICD-10-PCS (procedural categorization system) codes reflect outpatient procedures, ICD-10-CM (clinical modification) codes describe patients' conditions and diagnoses. The diagnosis code explains to the insurance payer why the service was rendered.

Local Coverage Determination (LCD): Determinations made by a contractor working with Medicare (MAC). An LCD may control specific codes. To avoid payment delays, it's crucial to frequently review LCDs to ensure your claims are accurate and complete before submitting them.

Medicare Administrative Contractor (MAC): A private health insurer that handles claims on behalf of Medicare enrollees is known as a Medicare Administrative Contractor (MAC).

Medicare Advantage Plans: Also known as Medicare Part C, these plans are an "all in one" alternative to traditional Medicare plans offered by private insurance companies.

Place of Service (POS): A two-digit code that designates the location where services were provided is called the "Place of Service" (POS).

Pre-Certification Number: The insurance provider will provide a pre-certification number indicating that the patient's services and treatment have been authorized; however, this does not ensure payment.

Prior Authorization Number: A number used to request specific treatments from the insurance payer. Make that the claim's prior authorization and referral numbers are accurate.

Provider Enrollment: Enrolling a provider in a commercial or government health insurance plan so they can be paid for the services they offer to patients is known as provider enrollment. For instance, the provider is deemed to be "in-network" once you have correctly registered with the insurance plan.

Remittance Advice Remark Codes (RARCs): Plans and issuers may use something called Remittance Advice Remark Codes (RARCs) to send information regarding claims to facilities and providers, as long as they comply with any applicable state laws. The RARC Committee has given its approval to the following RARCs in relation to the No Surprises Act, and these RARCs will become effective on March 1, 2022.

Rejected Claim: A claim is considered "rejected" when it has never been processed by either the clearinghouse, the insurance company, or the Centers for Medicare & Medicaid Services (CMS). There has been no "receipt" of the claim, and the adjudication (decision-making) process has not been finalized.

Revenue Cycle Management (RCM): Revenue Cycle Management Managing provider registration and credentialing, confirming eligibility and benefits, processing claims, posting payments, and generating revenue are all financial processes handled by a full RCM. To gather, manage, and collect patient service revenue, RCM and optometric billing services collaborate with your medical clearinghouse to expedite and simplify administrative and clinical tasks.

Secondary Insurance: After the original insurance has made a payment, the patient's secondary insurance covers some deductibles, co-pays, and co-insurance.

Superbill: A list of the services a patient receives from a healthcare provider used by those providers. The healthcare provider sends a paper or electronic claim to payers with the Superbill for payment.

Telehealth: Telehealth refers to remote non-clinical services.

Telemedicine: Clinical services delivered remotely.

Term Date: When an insurance policy expires, or a subscriber's or dependent's insurance coverage ends.

Third-Party Administrator (TPA): A third-party administrator (TPA) is a business that manages other claims administration services or processes insurance claims on behalf of healthcare providers.

Third-Party Payer: An organization that pays medical claims on behalf of the insured is a third-party payer, such as an insurance company, a government agency, an HMO, or an employer.

Type of Service (TOS): The Type of Service (TOS) field specifies the type of service rendered.

Unbundling: Unbundling is the practice of healthcare providers submitting several CPT treatment codes for a patient when only one is necessary.

Charges that are considered to be "Usual, Customary, and Reasonable" (UCR). The smallest amount of money that an insurance company is required to pay out in response to a claim being filed. Additionally, the UCR is the highest price that the majority of providers are all

owed to charge for particular medical services (depending on the service and geographic location).Write-Off or Adjustment Amount: A contractual adjustment is the amount that the insurance carrier has agreed to accept from the provider in order for them to continue to be a participating provider. A "write off" refers to the portion of the patient's bill that cannot be collected for any number of reasons.

Chapter 8: Is Medical Billing and Coding as Hard as it Seems?

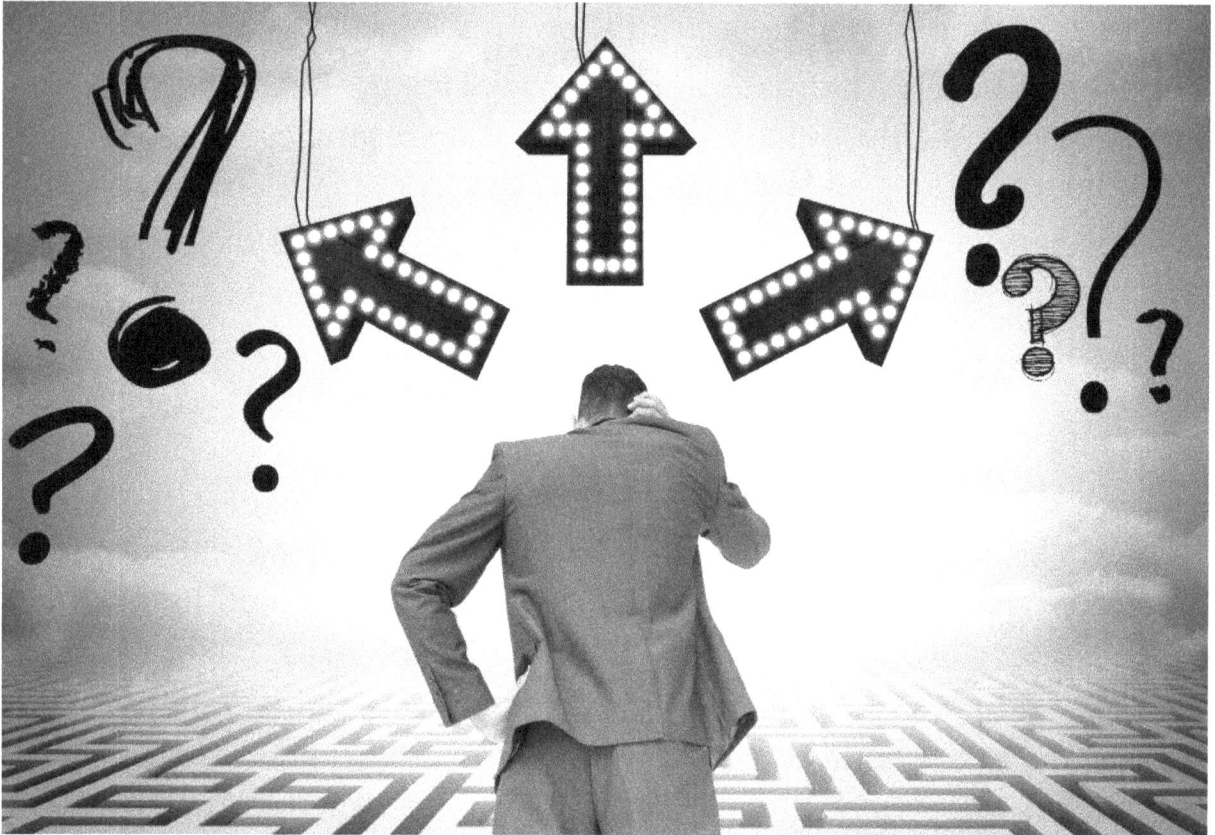

The need for healthcare providers in every area of the industry is expanding quickly along with the demand for healthcare services. These professionals are experiencing a boom in employment, including nurses, doctors, radiologists, and medical coders. At the same time, we are aware of these professions' complexity and unique demands. Healthcare personnel must deliver cutting-edge treatments and assist in caring for complex human problems. Medical billers and coders, for example, who do not deal directly with patients, face demands and tensions at work.

Is medical billing and coding challenging at the moment? Medical coding is the ideal option if you want to have a significant career on the administrative side of the healthcare industry. You can feel scared by the job's requirements, nevertheless. That is typical. After all, medical coders and billers deal with data daily.

Medical coders are in charge of gathering information from patient records and converting it into an international, alphanumeric code that other medical personnel and systems may utilize. Medical billers then use these codes to create insurance claims and guarantee that healthcare providers get paid for their services.

These professionals need abilities in detail orientation, data organization, memorization, and communication because of the nature of their work, which can sound like a long list to those just starting. But how challenging are medical billing and coding? If you get ready in advance, it doesn't have to be.

Is it Hard to Become a Medical Biller or Coder?

While occasionally challenging, medical billing and coding are by no means impossible.

Medical billing and coding are professions in the healthcare industry that require education and expertise. In other words, it will require a lot of effort. It takes time to improve as a medical coder or biller. This is so that you can understand the codes and classification systems used in the sector, which are essential for success. You must be proficient in using business software to charge patients and code information.

However, medical billing and coding strategies can come naturally to you if you enjoy learning. It's possible that with the proper education and work experience, you can master your field in a couple of months. In less than 18 months—faster than any other curriculum—Goodwin University's medical billing and coding certificate program assists students in becoming trained, certified, and employed in the profession. You will graduate from the program knowledgeable about the following:

- processing claims for health insurance
- examining patient records and medical records
- Medical procedure and diagnosis coding accuracy, including an understanding of CPT-4, ICD-10-CM, and HCPCS
- keeping track of risk withholds, deductibles, coinsurance, and copayments
- HIPAA guidelines

Having an effective dialogue with the larger healthcare team

Industry professionals that will assist you in learning the ropes are teaching the curriculum at Goodwin. They enjoy what they do, just like many medical billers and coders do! Although there are difficulties in medical billing and coding, there is a high level of job satisfaction. Medical records technicians, such as billers and coders, are ranked seventh among the top 30 positions in the healthcare support industry by U.S. News. Their work-life balance is strong, and they are more flexible than ordinary people. Working remotely makes life easier for many medical billers and coders. The complexity of the job, which determines how stressed-out medical billers and coders are, was also evaluated as being below average in the survey.

Don't Be Afraid of Medical Billing and Coding

Be confident even though this professional path requires classification and data processing. You won't ever be pushed into the deep end as a beginning medical biller and coder. Your training program of choice will guarantee that you possess the abilities and knowledge required to begin a career in the area. You can also be sure of the following as you start your new position:

- Your codebook is always available. Knowing all the medical codes takes time because so many of them exist. Your codebook may be the finest resource if you have a query.
- Technology for medical billing and coding is user-friendly. For you to perform this crucial role, industry software is created to be intuitive. You will do well if you have a foundational understanding of computers and formal training in the software you use.
- If you have finished a training course, you will be prepared. Programs in medical billing and coding, like the one offered by Goodwin, are made to position you for professional success. They will teach you health science fundamentals and the technical abilities required to decipher medical terminology, type computer code, and bill people. Additionally, a college-level curriculum will provide you with practical experience with various technologies so you can apply that knowledge

on your first day of work.

Medical Billing and Coding are Rewarding

A medical billing and coding career can be the right choice for you if you have a strong desire to serve people and a talent for details and data. This very fulfilling career enables you to influence the more significant healthcare industry. Healthcare professionals wouldn't be paid for their labor if medical billers and coders weren't there to process patient information correctly.

Medical coding and billing job might also entail a growth-oriented learning process. You will improve in your position as you gain more experience in the sector and face more difficulties at work. The better prepared you are to meet the challenges ahead, the more you will comprehend what problems can come your way and what each specific code implies. As they expand their expertise and experience, medical coders and billers have the opportunity to advance within the industry and take on new roles, such as health information managers, hospital coding managers, managers of medical and health services, and others.

Are Medical Billing and Coding Classes Hard to Complete?

We discussed the advantages of a healthy work-life balance for medical billers and coders, but what about medical billing and coding training? Is managing these college classes, a job, and family responsibilities challenging? Is it unattainable?

No, is the response. There are adaptable medical and billing programs available, prepared to assist you in moving forward in your career. You can choose classes that fit your schedule because Goodwin's medical billing and coding programs are offered daily and evening. You can select the best delivery method for you by choosing between on-campus and online options for courses.

Chapter 9: Pros and Cons of Being a Medical Biller and Coder

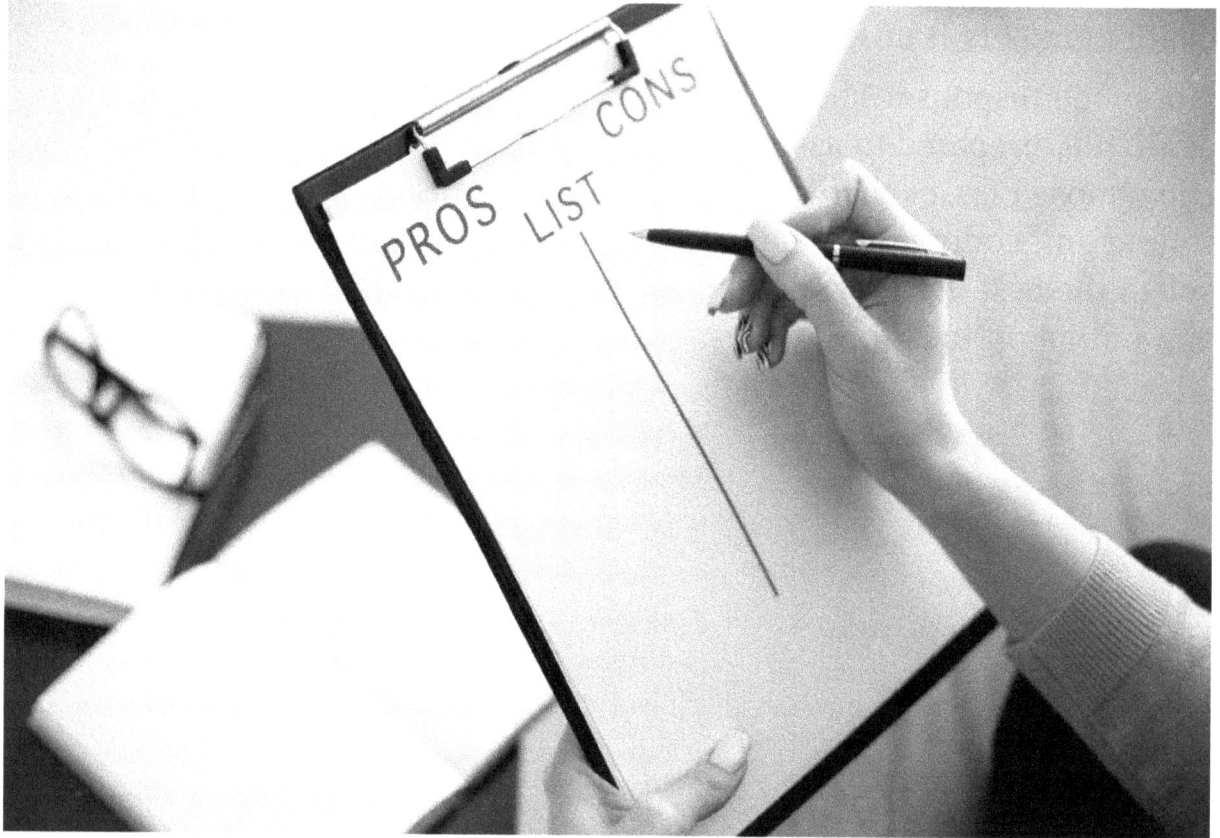

Cons

1. To be eligible for training programs, you must possess a high school diploma or GED.

You require a general education development degree or a high school diploma to qualify for medical and billing training programs (GED). You will be working with reasonably precise medical terminology, which is crucial. Thanks to the knowledge you acquire in high school, you will have the language and math abilities necessary to thrive in a medical billing and coding training program. This means that if you have not completed high school or your GED, you do not meet the qualifications to enroll in a medical billing and coding training program.

2. You must complete an accredited training program.

You must complete an official training course to work as a medical biller and coder. You can enroll in a certificate, diploma, or associate degree program. You can find training programs by consulting community colleges, technical schools, universities, hospitals, and other institutions that offer courses related to healthcare. The required training curriculum to become a medical biller and coder will take anywhere from 7 to 24 months to complete, depending on the type of institution you choose.

3. You need to be certified.

After finishing your training program, you must become certified to work as a medical biller and coder. A test is required to become certified. You must pass two certification exams to be a medical biller and coder. The first is the Certified Professional Coder (CPC) exam, and the second is the Registered Health Information Technician exam (RHIT). I genuinely hope you can pass these tests because if not, you'll have wasted your time and money.

4. You must update your certification.

Depending on the accrediting authority, one disadvantage of working as a medical biller and coder is that you might need to renew your certification every two to three years. Some people wonder if it will be worth it. This typically happens due to the requirement for continuing education hours to renew (CEUs). Because they can't "set it and forget" as they can in other occupations, some people find this tedious.

5.   There will be a considerable amount of new coding to learn.

As a medical biller and coder, you will be expected to learn a sizable number of ICD codes, and if new ones are added, you will also need to know those. This procedure must be repeated yearly because new ICD codes are introduced. There are now about 14,000 different ICD-9 code variations. ICD-10 now has over 110,000 unique codes. You are achieving total mastery over them.

6.   It is your responsibility to stay informed about any updates.

Medical billers and coders must keep up with any advancements in coding software. When coding some ICD-10 or CPT codes, improper information recognition could lead to severe issues. A recent modification to the ICD-10 code for the Ebola virus is an excellent illustration of this. Due to how recently it had been issued, only a small portion of medical billers and coders were familiar with the new code. Private health insurance firms responded by accusing those who omitted to update their software or failed to learn the code of submitting erroneous principles on behalf of their patients.

7.   Computer proficiency is a requirement.

Your duties as a medical coder and biller will frequently need you to use a computer. It is essentially your work tool. You won't be able to do your job and will almost likely feel more stressed since you don't know how to operate a computer.

8.   The possibility of developing carpal tunnel syndrome exists.

You risk developing carpal tunnel syndrome, one of the main drawbacks of being a medical biller and coder. Carpel tunnel syndrome is among the most typical ailments that medical billers and coders can experience. When the medial nerve, which passes through the wrist, becomes compressed, it causes carpal tunnel syndrome causes tingling or numbness in the hands. This condition can be excruciatingly uncomfortable and frustrating for medical coders and billers. If you experience this syndrome, you must change careers or work through the pain.

9.   The majority of your working day will be spent seated.

You will be seated at a desk all day if you work as a medical biller and coder. It is unhealthy to sit for such a long period. You spend the entire day working on charts, entering data, and conducting research while seated in front of a computer. This may result from numerous health issues, such as type 2 diabetes, cancer, obesity, heart disease, and blood clots.

10.   You won't make much money at your entry-level job.

The entry-level compensation for medical billers and coders is not particularly profitable, so keep that in mind as you consider the benefits and drawbacks of the profession. An hourly wage of $13.85 per hour, or roughly $28,800 per year, is what you may anticipate earning if you are just starting in the field. In some states, that is barely even minimum wage.

11.   You will frequently interact with outside parties.

Dealing with other parties regularly is one of the most significant drawbacks of being a medical biller and coder. These third parties may include employers, insurance providers, and government initiatives. These third companies often give you the runaround when you try to bill a claim or confirm benefits for a patient. You feel frustrated since you are in charge of obtaining accurate benefit information.

12.   Working as a medical coder and biller can be demanding.

Medical billing and coding can be a demanding profession. Stress can be too much to take at times. Even the most demanding people can crack under such intense pressure. Stress can negatively impact your mental and physical health if you do not learn how to manage it. Anxiety at work may hurt your connections.

13.   Working from home might be isolating.

It would help if you weighed several considerations while weighing the benefits and drawbacks of working remotely as a medical coder and biller. The solitude that comes with working from home is one of them. You can experience extreme loneliness. If you are not careful, the seclusion could negatively impact your mental health. When comparing the benefits and drawbacks of working remotely, it is essential to consider the absence of human contact outside your house.

Pros

1. A college education is not necessary to pursue this line of work.

After completing a relatively brief education and certification program, you can launch your career as a medical biller and coder. This is among the most significant advantages associated with working in this industry. Depending on the program you select, it could take anywhere from seven to twenty-four months to complete it. This indicates that you will be able to enter the workforce and begin producing money in a relatively short time following graduating from high school or obtaining your GED. To enter specific fields within the healthcare industry, you must complete several years of college after graduating from high school.

2. You have the option of finishing your training online.

Training for a career as a medical biller and coder can be finished online, which is one of the profession's many perks. You are free to complete your training anytime or night if you can learn online, which is one of the many advantages of having this capability. You can get it done whenever you have some spare time, such as before or after work, on the weekends, or any other day of the week. Training that is completed online will give you a great lot of flexibility to work around. It is also much simpler to continue your activity while learning online. Learning in a classroom could pique your attention at first, but after the first few weeks, boredom might set in, and you might find yourself skipping classes. Nothing truly changes when learning online; there is no need to travel, find parking, and sit in a classroom, so there is no need to lose interest. Because there is no need to do any of these things, there is no need to change.

3. Compared to the costs associated with training for other jobs, yours is a relatively inexpensive option.

Compared to the training required for other jobs, the amount of education you will need to become certified as a medical biller and coder is not that extensive. The amount necessary to finish a program might range from one thousand to three thousand dollars. In comparison to other types of work, that is nothing at all. As an illustration, the cost is significantly lower than that of becoming an electrician, which can range anywhere from $7,000 to $15,000. This is encouraging information for anyone who has an interest in working in the field of medical billing and coding.

4. There is scope for professional development.

Moving up the career ladder quickly is one of the many benefits of working in the medical billing and coding industry. After obtaining expertise in your discipline, you will have the opportunity to work in various fields, including practice management, medical auditing, compliance, clinical documentation improvement, education, and more. Some individuals who work in the medical billing and coding industry become consultants. They may concentrate on one particular kind of billing, such as electronic transactions or cardiology billing, as their primary area of expertise. While some full-time consultants establish a base of loyal clients and travel to work on multiple accounts, others remain in one location and focus on building that clientele. Advancing in your career may allow you to earn a higher wage.

5. You have the option of working from home.

Working from home is one of the primary perks of being a medical biller and coder, and it's also one of the most significant advantages. Those who do not wish to leave their children or pets alone at home throughout the day have the distinct advantage of using this tremendous benefit. It is also helpful for people who live in areas with a lot of snow and where it is impossible to get out of your driveway to go to work because of the snow. Working from home will also make it possible for you to finish all the duties that need to be done each day while still allowing you time for a salary job.

6. It is not required that you interact with a large number of people.

You won't have to interact with many patients if you want to become a medical biller and coder. This is because the patient will never see you, and, in this day and age, the majority of co-payments and claims have to be made via the internet. You won't have to deal with other individuals face-to-face at all. The phone call is the sole possible means of communication between you.

7. You have the option of working as a self-employed independent contractor.

You will have the opportunity to operate on your own as an independent contractor if you choose a career in medical billing and coding. You will be able to work for any healthcare facility that requires your expertise after you become a self-employed independent contractor. The kinds of services that a facility needs to be billed are the ones that will establish the type of facility you work for. You get to choose your hours when you're an independent contractor, which is one of the perks of having your own business. Because there is no predetermined schedule, you can take on as much work as possible.

8. You are flexible about where you can get a job.

You will have the option to work in various situations if you choose a career as a medical biller and coder. Billers and coders in the medical field can find employment with health insurance companies, hospitals, medical practices, rehabilitation centers, long-term care institutions, and even independent professional billing businesses, amongst other places. This is wonderful since it means that even if one setting does not work well for you, you have several more to experiment with until you find the one that works the best for you.

9. People are clamoring to work with you.

One of the many benefits of working in the medical billing and coding industry is you won't have to relocate anytime soon. You may expect to be in demand for a very long time as a medical biller and coder for a considerably more extended period than the typical individual would anticipate from a job. Because there are not enough people qualified to fill these positions, it is not rare for skilled coders to continue working well into their seventies. You have a lot of work stability in addition to the fact that you are in high demand. Because you will have so many alternatives available, you will be in a position to make essential choices for yourself and your family.

10. You are not restricted in where you work.

Working practically anywhere is one of the primary benefits of working as a medical biller and coder. Because there is a demand for workers in this field across the entirety of the United States, you won't have to move to keep your employment unless you're dying for a change of pace. You won't have any trouble finding work in a physician's office, medical facility, or hospital; you may even work for one of the several businesses that focus on medical billing and coding.

11. You will finally make a very comfortable livelihood for yourself

When considering the benefits and drawbacks of a medical billing and coding career, it is essential to remember that you will eventually earn a good living. Although your starting income of $28,800 per year is not ideal, if you demonstrate exceptional performance, you may be able to increase your earnings to an average of $48,270 per year in the future. A boost in pay of just over $20,000 is immensely satisfying.

12. You can have a versatile work schedule.

Working as a medical biller and coder allows you to enjoy the benefits of a flexible work schedule. Monday through Friday is the standard schedule for a workweek for someone responsible for medical billing and coding. On the other hand, some jobs allow employees to determine their plans for the week so long as they accomplish all of the responsibilities. Now, if you work from home, you can adjust your schedule to accommodate whatever is going on in your life. This will be possible since you will have more flexibility.

13. Your employment will provide you with some enjoyable benefits.

Several enticing benefits come along with working as a medical biller and coder. You and your family will be eligible for health benefits, receive paid vacation time and additional time off, and have the opportunity to work in a field you are passionate about.

Deciding to pursue a career in medical billing and coding is significant. It will impact your future, the satisfaction you derive from your profession, and even the health of others around you. Billers and coders in the medical industry are essential components of the healthcare system. Your employers and your patients will benefit greatly from the valuable service you give, as it will save them time, money, and other resources. Being a professional in medical billing comes with several advantages. However, there is also the possibility of negatives; this article on the benefits and drawbacks of working as a medical biller and coder has highlighted some of them so that you are aware of what you can anticipate if you choose to pursue this line of work. I hope that the top 13 benefits and drawbacks of working as a medical biller and coder you have just read will assist you in deciding whether or not you should pursue this career path.

Chapter 10: medical coding mistakes that could cost you

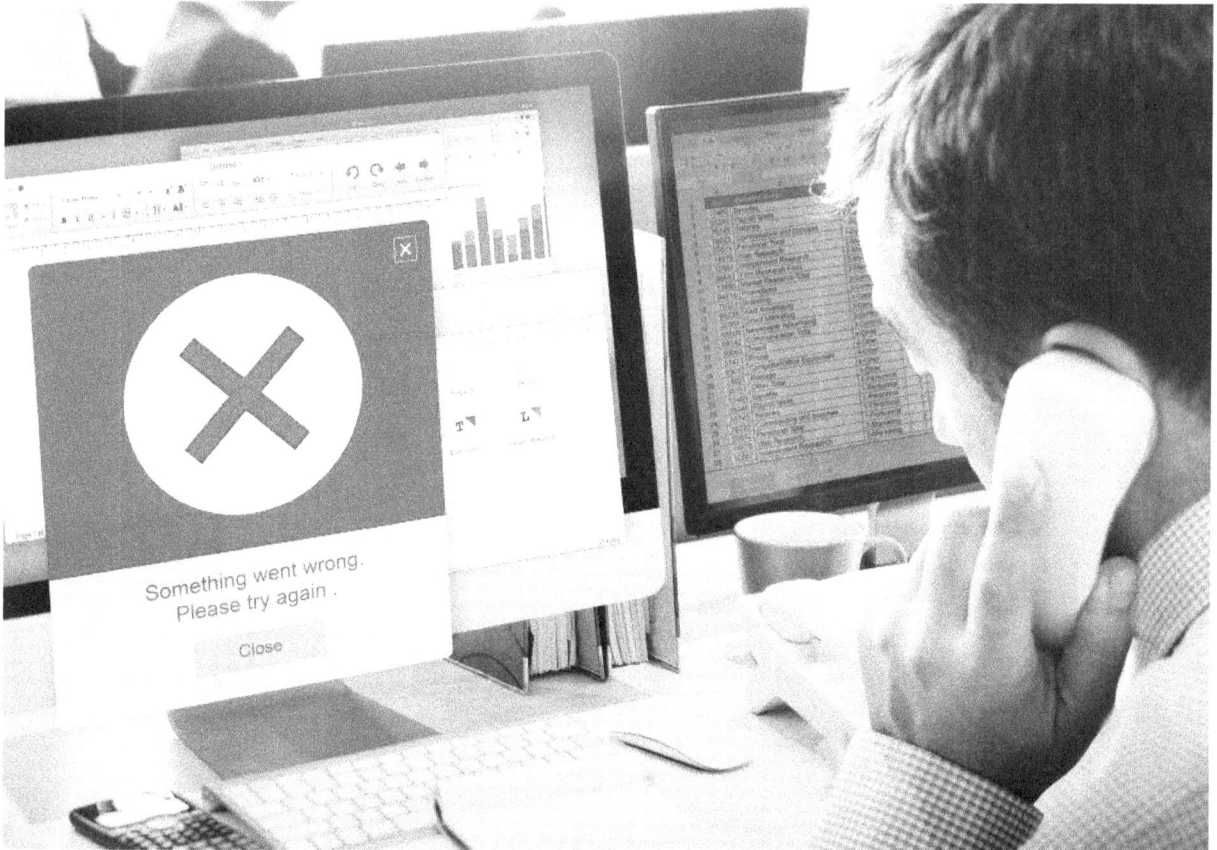

The regrettable instances of fraudulent or abusive medical billing practices have been uncovered through audits conducted by government and private insurers. While you should be compensated for the medical services you render, staying out of legal hot water and keeping your practice thriving requires that you avoid unethical billing methods.

Amendments to the Current Procedural Terminology Codebook

The American Medical Association's (AMA) efforts to streamline paperwork and reduce note bloat are ongoing. If you want to know more about the continuing efforts to improve CPT, subscribe immediately.

Medical coding mistakes can be divided into two primary groups: fraud and abuse.

The former type involves dishonesty on purpose. In the latter case, "the fabrication was an innocent mistake, but representative," as stated in the AMA's Principles of CPT® Coding, Ninth Edition. "for a more sophisticated service than was performed owing to misunderstanding the coding system," the literature explains, is an example of misuse.

The American Medical Association (AMA) maintains several tools to assist in correctly billing for medical services and procedures using the Current Procedural Terminology (CPT) and Healthcare Common Procedure Coding System (HCPCS) code sets.

Coding resources from the recognized leader in the CPT code set can be found at the AMA Online Store. The Codebook, Online Coding Subscriptions, Data Files, and Coding Packages are available here.

Read on for examples of the most frequent mistakes when classifying medical records.

I am taking codes apart.

It is utilizing a single code that accounts for payment for all aspects of a procedure wherever possible is preferable. Unbundling refers to assigning different CPT codes to distinct elements of an operation to maximize reimbursement or clarify the nature of the service provided.

Upcoding.

You're a doctor who works in a field like oncology, where you regularly see patients who present multiple challenges. As a result, regardless of the patient's natural state, you report the most extensive evaluation and management (E/M) service possible. It is essential to correctly say the degree of E/M code based on the patient's condition rather than relying solely on your specialty (this is not always upcoding).

Of course, there are instances of blatant upcoding fraud. This should serve as a cautionary tale. Due partly to upcoding, one psychiatrist was fined $400,000 and indefinitely banned from Medicare and Medicaid participation. Instead of meeting with patients for 15 minutes at a time to check their meds, he billed for 30- or 60-minute sessions.

Multi-code reporting without first checking for NCCI corrections.

The National Correct Coding Initiative was established by the Centers for Medicare & Medicaid Services to assist with monitoring Medicare

Part B claims and preventing improper payments through the use of accurate coding practices. Prepayment edits are "reached by examining every pair of codes billed for the same patient on the same service date by the same provider to see if an alteration exists in the NCCI," as stated in the AMA's wording. One of the codes is rejected if an NCCI edit is performed. NCCI modifications will often also include a list of CPT modifiers that can be utilized to bypass the edit and submit the claim. Some situations expressly forbid the employment of any qualifiers to overrule an adverse ruling.

As an illustration, suppose you do both the excision of a lesion and the subsequent healing of the skin on the same service day. However, according to the CPT coding guidelines, minor repairs must be coded as part of the excision codes. Suppose the repair was done in a location other than where the lesion was excised. In that case, however, it is acceptable to bill for both the excision and the restoration, with a modifier to alert the payer that the two procedures were distinct.

It is incorrectly attaching modifiers or omitting necessary ones.

A scenario similar to the one described may include adding the modifier 50, Bilateral Procedure, to a procedure code that already describes bilateral service.

Increased Procedural Services is excessive use of modifier 22.

If the procedure takes longer than usual, you should capture that fact.

Here's an illustration: you operate on a highly overweight patient and remove a neck crease. Obesity increases the difficulty of the excision. Adding modifier 22 to the removal report code can show the increased complexity of the service in these cases.

Incorrect recording of the time-based infusion and hydration codes.

Coders in the medical field can't get paid for their work unless they correctly charge for these services. There are additional complexities with services that span more than one day.

In this case, the patient receives continuous intravenous hydration from 11 p.m. to 2 a.m. In that situation, the two doses shouldn't be reported together as a single constant infusion but rather as two independent initials (96374) sequential doses (96376).

Codes for injections being misreported.

Avoid reporting several code units and write a single code for the sessions during which the injections occur.

I was not having the proper paperwork when reporting an unlisted code.

If you need to bill for a service using a code that isn't on the list, you must ensure you have all the proper paperwork.

How to Prevent These Errors Occurring

Coding is the single most essential safeguard against fraud in medical billing. Medical coders and billers should thoroughly understand the medical procedures they may encounter. That includes each year's crop of brand-new codes introduced with the yearly refresh. Therefore, educating people is crucial so that medical billing mistakes are avoided. To succeed in the competitive medical billing and coding field, it's not enough to know the ins and outs; you need to be certified. Without software packages that contain reminders and checklists for training and keeping up with the required codes, there is more possibility for errors in hospitals and doctors' offices.

Utilizing a claims clearinghouse is yet another method for reducing the likelihood of billing and coding errors in the medical industry. Before being forwarded to the appropriate party, this clearinghouse will do an error check; if any are found, the claim will be returned to you for correction. Doing so can help your office run more smoothly by cutting down on mistakes and alleviating some stress.

Finally, the most excellent way to avoid medical billing and coding mistakes is through open lines of communication. To complete the essential paperwork for the billing department, doctors must coordinate with patients and nurses. In addition, there must be no leaks in the lines of communication between departments. Correct data entry at the front desk allows for cross-checking patient records with billing records to prevent double or incorrect billing. To work efficiently, all doctors and staff must have a solid understanding of the coding regulations to avoid costly and time-consuming mistakes.

Chapter 11: Ten Ways to Ensure Precise Medical Billing And Coding

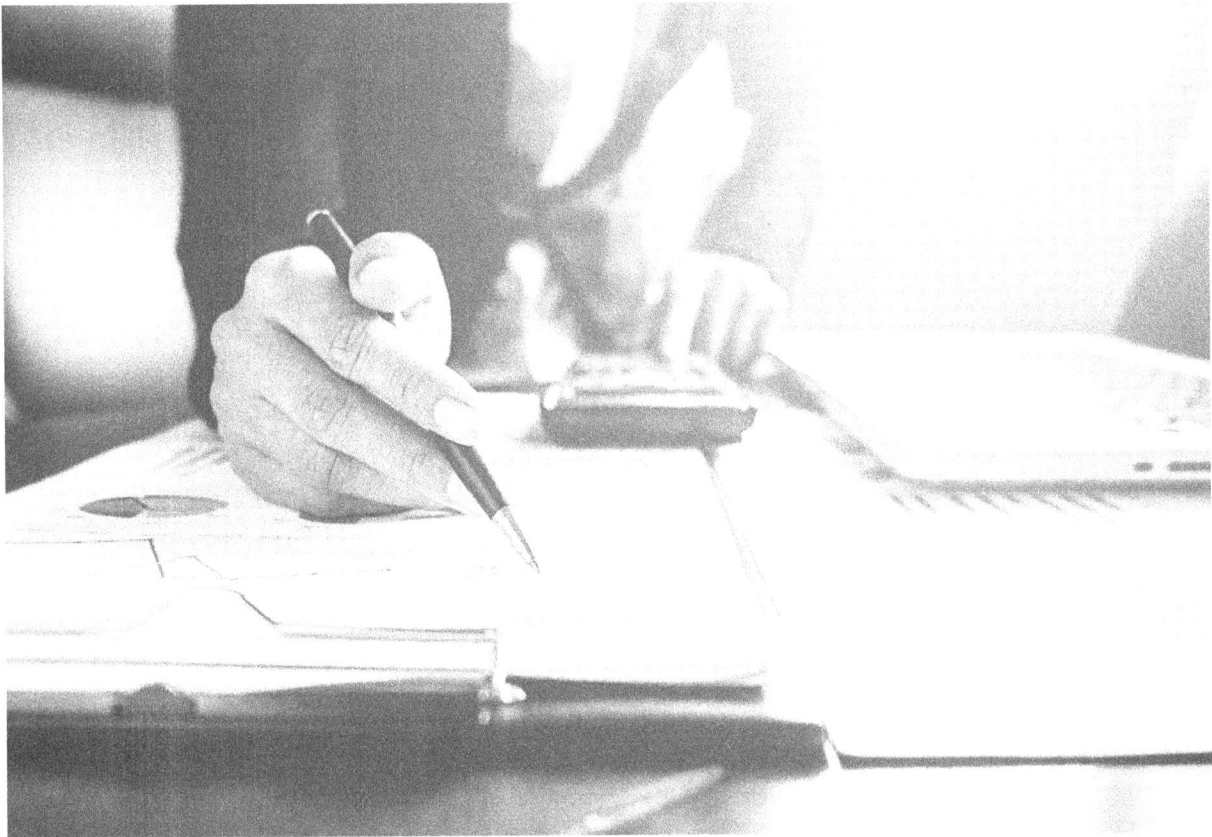

Several issues might arise from incorrect medical coding and billing. Denied or partially paid claims are expensive not just in terms of dollars and cents but also in terms of time, delayed payments, lower quality patient care, angry patients, reputational damage, and, worst-case scenario, audits and fines that can put the practice at danger.

Experts predict that as much as 80% of all medical invoices contain inaccuracies, meaning that 80% of claims will be denied. And the outcome is the same: no reimbursement, whether due to insufficient proof, double billing, or a simple error in the account number.

Don't let frequent coding and billing mistakes derail your efforts to improve accuracy.

Aim for Precision.

Incorrect payments and claims denials can be avoided if preventative measures are taken. Look out for these ten mistakes when submitting a claim:

The cost that isn't going to be reimbursed:

Billing for an item the patient's insurance doesn't cover is the most common billing mistake. To avoid this, it is recommended to check coverage before providing the service. If you have questions about whether your Medicare claim will be paid, you should review Chapter 16: General Exclusions in the Medicare Benefit Policy Manual.

Data inaccuracies or omissions:

A denial will occur if the necessary patient, provider, or insurance information is either missing or entered incorrectly. Despite its apparent simplicity, this mistake is more likely to happen when multiple personnel is responsible for processing a single claim. Verify the correctness of all names, insurance ID numbers, and other identifying information before submitting a claim, regardless of whether you are the first or last person to touch the file.

When two or more service providers seek payment (or payment) for the same service, this is known as double billing (or duplicate billing). It is critical to check whether or not a service has been billed for previously, as doing so might lead to accusations of fraud and sanctions from regulatory bodies if it happens too often.

The term "unbundling" describes the practice of separately itemizing costs for what should be grouped in a single category. Intentionally or unintentionally, unbundling services incorrectly to increase reimbursement constitutes fraud. If you want to know which codes are packaged and whether or not unbundling is allowed, you should look at the revisions made by the National Correct Coding Initiative.

Up-coding is erroneously using a code to represent a more severe diagnosis or treatment to receive a higher reimbursement rate. To prevent potential legal repercussions, providers should avoid engaging in this conduct, violating the federal False Claims Act.

Failure to record the full scope of services/procedures ("under-coding") does not protect a practice from denials and audits. The method loses money when doctors under-code, and patients may suffer unfavorable consequences if inaccurate information is reported.

Under-documentation occurs when a physician fails to provide sufficient details about patient interaction, leaving the coder unable to assign correct codes. The absence of "medical need" is commonly cited as denial in such cases. If you feel your doctor's notes do not adequately reflect the level of care being billed, it is essential to discuss this with them to understand better.

Using modifier 22 too often:

Addendum 22 Extended Procedural Support is meant just for surgical operations and not for use with E/M service codes. Modifier 22 can be added to a CPT® code "where the work required to perform a service is much greater than generally required," according to the CPT® guidelines. However, the meaning of "significantly greater" is ambiguous, leading various service providers to adopt their definitions. Be ready to provide documentation if asked to do so by payers, and make sure to have it on hand to back up your use of this modification.

Misuse of out-of-date code:

Changes to code sets following the annual January 1 refresh are usual. Ensure you're using the latest up-to-date codes when submitting claims by checking for updates frequently throughout the year.

Prior incurred expenses:

For this reason, it is always futile to submit a claim for work completed prior to the insurance policy's effective date. Check the patient's insurance status before each appointment.

Conclusion

Coders and billers in the medical industry are highly esteemed contributors to patient care. Their efforts keep the business afloat financially and free up professional personnel to give each patient their full attention. As a medical billing or coding expert, you can work remotely from the comfort of your own home.

There are many openings and job security in healthcare because of the growing elderly population and many current healthcare workers' retirement.

Because of the widespread prevalence of healthcare institutions, you can choose desirable locations and work environments to pursue a career in the healthcare industry. After entering the field, you will have several opportunities to further your career through management or in a more direct caregiving role. Most importantly, medical coders' and billers' work can directly impact patients' health and well-being.

A career in medical billing and coding calls for meticulous planning and execution. Working in medical billing and coding could be an excellent fit for you if you are a detail-oriented, organized, and capable multitasker.

Candidates also need to be at ease in an office atmosphere, as they will spend a great deal of time in front of a computer and handling patient records. Knowing or being ready to learn a medical language is crucial. A willingness to learn new things is essential for workers in this industry, as they must adapt to the ever-evolving procedures and coding requirements.

Medical coding and billing career is a fantastic option if you fit this profile.

www.ingramcontent.com/pod-product-compliance
Lightning Source LLC
Chambersburg PA
CBHW081822200326
41597CB00023B/4350